Patient
Self-Determination
in
Long-Term Care

Marshall B. Kapp, JD, MPH, was educated at Johns Hopkins University (B.A.), George Washington University (J. D. With Honors), and Harvard University (M.P.H.). In his positions with the Health Care Financing Administration and the New York State Office of Federal Affairs, he gained substantial experience in health regulation generally, and aging in particular. Since August 1980, he has been a faculty member in the School of Medicine at Wright State University, Dayton, Ohio, where he is a Professor in the Department of Community Health and Director of the WSU Office of Geriatric Medicine and Gerontology. He holds an adjunct faculty appointment at the University of Dayton School of Law. In addition to being admitted to practice law in a number of state and federal courts, he is also licensed as a Nursing Home Administrator in the District of Columbia. He is the author of a substantial number of published books, articles, and reviews. Dr. Kapp is a Fellow of the Gerontological Society of America.

Patient Self-Determination in Long-Term Care

Implementing the PSDA in Medical Decisions

Marshall B. Kapp, JD, MPH
Editor

•

The inaugural volume in the
Springer Series on Ethics, Law, and Aging

Series Editor: Marshall B. Kapp, JD, MPH

Springer Publishing Company

Cover and interior design by Holly Block

Springer Publishing Company, Inc.
536 Broadway
New York, NY 10012

94 95 96 97 98 / 5 4 3 2 1

Library of Congress Cataloging-in-Publication Data

Patient self-determination in long-term care : implementing the PSDA in medical decisions / Marshall B. Kapp, editor.
  p.   cm.
  Includes bibliographical references and index.
  ISBN 0-8261-8520-7
  1. Nursing home care—United States—Moral and ethical aspects.
2. Terminal care—United States—Decision making.   3. Patients—Legal status, laws, etc.—United States.   4. Informed consent (Medical law)—United States.   5. Right to die—Law and legislation—United States.   6. Aged—Long-term care—United States—Moral and ethical aspects.   7. Ethics committees.   I. Kapp, Marshall B.
RA997.P286   1994
362.1'6—dc20   94-17537
                                                                                      CIP

Printed in the United States of America

Chapter 7 is from "Liability Issues and Assessment of Decision-Making Capability in Nursing Home Patients" by M. B. Kapp, November 1990, *American Journal of Medicine*, © 1990 by Cahner's Publishing Company. Reprinted by permission.

Chapter 8 is from "State Statutes Limiting Advance Directives: Death Warrants or Life Sentences?" by M. B. Kapp, 1992, *Journal of the American Geriatrics Society, 40*, pp. 722–726. © 1992 by the American Geriatrics Society. Reprinted by permission.

Contents

v

Contributors

Sister Agnes M. Boes, RSM, is Director of Resident Services, Mission Services, and Continuous Quality Improvement at Mercy Sienna Woods, Dayton, Ohio. She holds Masters degrees in psychiatric nursing and in health services administration and was instrumental in establishing the Institutional Ethics Committee at Mercy Sienna Woods.

Monsignor Charles J. Fahey is Senior Associate, Third Age Center, Fordham University, a former President of the American Society on Aging, American Association of Homes for the Aging, and Catholic Charities, U.S.A.

Amy Marie Haddad, RN, PhD, C., is Associate Professor and Chair, Department of Administrative and Social Sciences, School of Pharmacy and Allied Health Professions, Creighton University. She is also a Faculty Associate in Creighton's Center for Health Policy and Ethics.

William Kavesh, MD, is Chair of the Division of Geriatrics, Albert Einstein Medical Center (Philadelphia). He is also a member of the faculty at Temple University School of Medicine.

Vernellia R. Randall, RN, MSN, JD, is Assistant Professor in the School of Law, University of Dayton. She is also an Assistant Voluntary Professor in the Department of Community Health, Wright State University School of Medicine. Prior to attending law school, she provided public health nursing services and served as an administrator for a statewide health program in Alaska.

Todd L. Sobol, MD, is an internist in private medical practice in Dayton, Ohio, an Assistant Clinical Professor, Department of Medicine, Wright State University School of Medicine, and Medical Director and Institutional Ethics Committee member at Covenant House in Dayton.

Acknowledgments

Every book is a team effort. This observation is especially true for this volume because it is based on a conference held on March 19, 1993 in Dayton, Ohio. I acknowledge with appreciation the efforts and cooperation of my co-sponsor Miami Valley Gerontology Council (with the Wright State University Office of Geriatric Medicine & Gerontology), with special thanks to Susan Hayes, Pam Fenn, Kenneth Daily, and their committee members. The administrative support of Margie Dean (Miami Valley Gerontology Council) and Christina DeWitt (Wright State University Office of Geriatric Medicine and Gerontology) in working out conference logistics was essential. Naturally, the enthusiastic participation and follow-through of conference speakers who contributed chapters to this volume was indispensable. As always, working with the staff of Springer Publishing—from initial conceptualization and organization through final production—was a professional and personal pleasure. Last, but not least, the financial support of the Thomas Fordham Foundation (Dayton) in subsidizing the conference upon which this book was built, is gratefully acknowledged.

Introduction

The amount of professional literature and popular press material published in the past decade regarding the topics of medical decision-making for seriously ill individuals and advance medical directives (including living wills and durable powers of attorney) is virtually overwhelming, even to professionals who regularly work in this arena. The avalanche of written words has become stronger since 1990, when the United States Congress enacted the Patient Self-Determination Act (PSDA) (Public Law No. 101–508, §§4206, 4751), which followed closely the Supreme Court's decision in *Cruzan v. Director, Missouri Department of Health*, 110 S. Ct. 2841 (1990).

Given a situation where one can barely keep up with copying and filing (let alone reading and digesting) the current literature on ethical and legal implications of initiating, continuing, withholding, and withdrawing life-sustaining medical treatments, it may fairly be asked if the world needs yet another contribution to the reading pile.

The hopeful answer represented by the current volume is in the affirmative. This is a front-burner issue for health care professionals today. The need for health care providers to develop and implement specific policies and procedures for addressing difficult choices about particular forms of medical intervention for particular patients has been underscored by the PSDA. This legislation imposes on nursing facilities and home care agencies (as well as hospitals, hospices, health maintenance organizations, and preferred provider organizations) a number of new obligations concerning informed consent, advance instruction and proxy directives, staff and community education, and other facets of medical decision-making for seriously ill and incompetent patients.

Although an enormous amount of attention has been devoted in the literature recently to how acute care hospitals—and in particular critical care units—should meet their obligations in this regard, relatively little attention and assistance has been directed toward nursing facilities, and almost none to home care agencies. Particularly in light of the interaction of the PSDA with the fairly new Omnibus Budget Reconciliation Act (OBRA) of 1987, requirements for both nursing facilities and home care providers and a spate of varied state laws on this subject, long-term care providers desperately need clear, practical advice on grappling with the legal and ethical challenges raised by the process of medical decision-making near the end of life. The present book is intended to fill this important gap.

Illustrations of the kind of questions that long-term care providers face in the 1990s include:

- Should provider policies specifically refer to specific religious or philosophical principles undergirding the provider's central mission?
- Should a provider's policy explicitly warn that the provider's commitment to specific religious or philosophical principles might negate patient or surrogate choices in certain matters (e.g., artificial nutrition and hydration)?
- Should a provider's policy contain a conscience clause excusing staff from participating in the implementation of treatment choices with which the staff member strongly disagrees?
- Should a provider's policy explicitly declare the provider's claimed right to transfer a patient for refusing recommended care or for demanding interventions that the provider believes would be futile?

- Should the provider have a separate written policy regarding such matters as artificial feeding and hydration or resuscitation and Do Not Resuscitate (DNR, or No Code) orders? Alternatively, should general medical treatment policies distinctly contain these issues?
- Should the provider's policy expressly state that the courts may be necessary (or mandatory) to resolve certain disputes?
- Should the provider's policy specifically guarantee (rather than rely on an implied understanding) that comfort measures will always be available?
- Should the provider's policy encourage mentally competent patients to execute advance directives, or should the provider just provide information and otherwise remain neutral?
- Should the provider's policy encourage a patient or surrogate to consult with an institutional ethics committee, an attorney, or a member of the clergy, and under what circumstances? Should the provider undertake to facilitate such consultation on the patient/surrogate's behalf?
- Under a provider's policy, should there be an Institutional Ethics Committee (IEC)? If so, what functions should the IEC perform?
- If case consultation is a function assigned to the IEC, who should have the right or authority to bring a case to the IEC—the patient, family members, or other surrogates, provider staff (all or only certain employees), attending physician, and/or outsiders?
- For any of these categories, should bringing a case to the IEC be mandatory? If so, in what situations?
- Should anyone, including the patient or attending physician, have the right or authority to veto IEC involvement in a case?
- Should the IEC take recorded votes in individual cases? Should the IEC operate by majority vote versus consensus versus discussion without any attempt to reach majority vote or consensus?
- If the IEC takes votes in particular cases, should the results be binding or advisory on the participants?
- Should IEC discussion in particular cases consist of all IEC members or a panel (of what size and composition?) ap-

pointed for each case? Should the IEC maintain a consultant list of persons outside IEC membership who might be
appointed to a panel in a specific case?
- What written records, if any, should the IEC create regarding its consultation in a particular case? Where should
these records be maintained and who should have access to
them? Should the patient's medical record indicate that the
IEC has been involved in the case?
- Should the IEC be organized as a committee of the Board of
Trustees or Board of Directors, of the organization's administration, or the provider's organized medical staff (if such
exists)?

These queries represent the sort of issues that contributors
of the ensuing chapters set out to tackle. This volume had its
genesis in a March 19, 1993, conference held in Dayton, Ohio
and cosponsored by the Wright State University School of
Medicine's Office of Geriatric Medicine and Gerontology and
the Miami Valley Gerontology Council. Over six hundred
people heard from nationally and locally prominent experts
in the theory and practice of enhancing patient self-determination in long-term care. Conference presentations have been
expanded, updated, edited for overall cohesiveness, and supplemented by additional material.

Monseigneur Charles Fahey's contribution sets the stage by
raising important and difficult issues about the moral implementation of a new law—the Patient Self-Determination Act—
that has raised high public expectations. He shows how ethics
involves questions of caring that cannot be resolved simply by
resorting to legislative language. He thoughtfully explicates
the ethical status and responsibility of all the stakeholders in
the long-term care decision-making environment: the patient,
professional caregivers, surrogate decisionmakers, and institutional administrators.

Next, Dr. William Kavesh concentrates on the physician's
special role as a participant in the interdisciplinary process
dealing humanely with medical decision-making situations in
long-term facilities and home care environments. Recommendations for optimizing the performance of physicians in ful-

filling this role are made both for physicians and for other professionals who work with them on long-term care interdisciplinary teams.

Dr. Todd Sobol and Sister Agnes Boes carefully analyze the potential and the pitfalls of utilizing various forms of Institutional Ethics Committees (IECs) in the nursing home setting. They discuss purposes and objectives, legal implications, the process of decision-making protocol development, policy-formulation issues, the role of IECs in education and case consultation, and various operational details entailed in creating and maintaining a productive long-term care IEC. Their chapter finishes with a foray into ethical problem-solving techniques.

In Chapter 4, nurse/ethicist Amy Haddad presents valuable advice to professionals involved in advance planning for medical choices with home care clients and their families. She articulately illustrates how implementation of the PSDA raises unique challenges in the home care setting, and how principles and processes may be transposed to this setting from hospitals and nursing homes only with the greatest of caution.

Next comes a chapter by attorney Marshall Kapp that explicates some of the chief ethical and legal wrinkles implicated by the orchestration of a home-based death. The advent of high-tech home care raises a variety of ethical and legal concerns, as the home environment moves from a place where treatment decisions made elsewhere are merely carried out to a place where decision-making itself happens.

In Chapter 6, Professor Vernellia Randall offers a provocative interpretation of the influence of a patient's race and ethnicity on the patient's reaction to the PSDA in a long-term care atmosphere. Sensitivity to these racial and ethnic factors is imperative for health care providers, administrators, and public policymakers who might otherwise tend to overgeneralize about patients in the quest for a single "solution" to the long-term care decision-making dilemma.

Chapter 7 examines the problem of trying to make working assessments about the decisional capacity of nursing home

residents, with specific attention to the often perverse influence of anxiety about liability on this assessment process.
The author addresses provider perceptions and their behavioral consequences, attempts to put liability risks into some
realistic perspective, and suggests workable risk-management
strategies and viable public-policy options.

The final chapter swims against the mainstream of most
current commentary on advance directives by condemning,
rather than praising, the majority of state legislation enacted
in the past decade dealing with instruction and proxy directives. Contemporary state advance directive statutes, which
tend to limit instead of expand individual treatment options,
are attacked here as: damaging autonomy; fostering confusion, uncertainty, and unpredictability; increasing rather
than diminishing the threat of litigation; discouraging time-
limited trials of potentially beneficial (but also potentially di-
sastrous) medical interventions; driving some desperate patients into the arms of suicide advocates; violating ethical
principles of distributive justice by misallocating precious resources; and fomenting general disrespect for the rule of law.
Practical guidelines for physicians are presented to cope with
the legislative quagmire.

This volume does not pretend, nor is it intended, to be a
simple how-to or technical instruction manual that nursing
facilities or home care agencies can facilely superimpose on
their own patients, families, staffs, and communities. A detailed, inflexible template of this sort would be a mirage,
given the unique missions, contexts, strengths, and limitations that characterize each different long-term care
provider.

However, fundamental ethical and legal principles do exist
to guide and aid individual providers toward the development, application, evaluation, and improvement of policies
and procedures that honor patient autonomy while respecting other, potentially competing interests. We have tried here
to identify, reflect upon, and suggest the application of these
principles as a framework for action. If this book further sen-
sitizes those who have the difficult but indispensable social

role of providing long-term health and human services to dependent persons, to the principles and processes likely to foster good ethical and legal treatment of patients (at a point
when they are most vulnerable to abuse or neglect at the
hands of others), its addition to the burgeoning literature will
be justified indeed.

The Moral Aspects of the Patient Self-Determination Act

1

Monsignor Charles J. Fahey

THE CONTEXT

The latter part of the 20th century has seen the development of marvelous technologies and procedures which allow us to live longer, less painful, and more certain lives than persons at any other moment of history. We have unparalleled opportunities for education, recreation, cultural pursuits, and personal relationships. Even in instances of chronic illness or disability, pharmacological agents and prosthetic devices enable many people to live satisfying and productive lives.

However, all development, including that which wards off death, is ambiguous. Technological advances tend to be pressed into usage before we develop moral perspectives and social structures to utilize them in our service and that of the physical environment within which we live. Atomic energy and pesticides come to mind, just as do ventilators and imaging machines.

To some extent we have done away with "natural" death. Now we are challenged to reinvent the dying process in the light of late 20th-century values, culture, and technology.

1

Such an effort is particularly daunting to a society that is both pluralistic and given to an almost obsessive focus on privacy and individualism.

The Patient Self-Determination Act (PSDA) can be the occasion of enriching the dying experience by better integrating this reality into our everyday lives. However, if it is viewed merely as another bureaucratic, regulatory requirement to meet with a minimalist response, then it will be an opportunity lost; both individuals and society will be further impoverished.

It should come as no surprise that the Act should have been sponsored by Senators Danforth and Moynihan, since celebrated court cases in their home states (*Cruzan* in Missouri and *O'Connor* in New York) illustrated our ineptness as a society in making decisions about and attending to the dying process. However, the very legislation, as well intentioned and useful as it could be, illustrates the limitations and even the clumsiness of law when it touches this part of the human journey.

Neither the fact situation nor the decisions in the cases need be discussed here in detail. However, it should be noted that in two different jurisdictions the loved ones of two women who in all likelihood would have been long dead in another era were confronted by professional and legal systems that in effect distorted the dying process. In each instance, professionals and institutions felt compelled to use the legal system to decide their course of action, instituting a long, expensive, cumbersome, and apparently painful psychological process which ultimately reached the highest court in their respective jurisdictions. In the instance of Nancy Cruzan, the case was decided by the Supreme Court of the United States (*Cruzan v. Director, Missouri Department of Health*, 110 S.Ct. 2841 (1990)). In both instances, the state courts required high levels of evidence indicating that the patient's explicit wishes were that life-sustaining measures be removed in such circumstances; this in the face of testimony of attentive family members who testified that each woman would not have wished to have the dying process prolonged under the circumstances.

The Patient Self-Determination Act is something of a legal anomaly. Ordinarily, matters affecting life and death are matters of state jurisdiction. This Act seized upon the only tools that seemed available at the federal level to begin to address issues raised in these and similar cases, namely, Medicare and Medicaid reimbursement to providers. The Act's intent is twofold: to encourage providers to be sensitive to advance directives, and to encourage individuals to execute such documents. Ironically, in identifying providers who should inquire about advance directives, it omits that provider who is in the best position to deal with the subject, namely the doctor, and instead addresses itself to those that, at best, are modestly equipped, namely, medical institutions. While a visit to a physician would seem to be one of the occasions when a discussion of advance directives would be appropriate, the entry into a formal care program, often with attendant confusion, pain and concern, is just the opposite.

SURROGATE DECISIONMAKING

An advance directive is a means by which a person can maintain some control over health decisions, even in the face of compromised mental ability. State legislatures have developed such instruments to enable persons to exercise moral agency in their health affairs even when they become mentally incapacitated. Such statutes are based on the premise that persons wish to exercise such control, and their wishes can be expressed in writing, through a surrogate, or through some combination of the two. (This premise, by the way, is by no means self-evident.)

There is general agreement among scholars that personal integrity involves moral agency. A person has the primary, if not altogether exclusive, moral and legal right to make decisions in regard to his or her own health care. Advance directives are a means to extend that moral agency to a time and place when and where a person may not have the capacity to express his or her own wishes. They allow the identification of a person, in the instance of the durable power of attorney, who will make the person's wishes known or, in the instance of the "living will," the kind of treatment the person would have wanted were he or she able to express a preference.

In my judgment, living wills are a poor second to health care proxies or durable powers of attorney. They have two structural weaknesses. It is virtually impossible to anticipate the circumstances both of the patient and of medicine at the time such might be utilized. Secondly, it at least implicitly removes medical decisions from the domain of a friend or family member. Such decisions cannot be made by a computer or a piece of paper but by a human being with moral sensitivities. A living will does not call for a friend or relative to be involved in the original decisions about suffering, life and death, nor does it identify the person the prospective patient would want to accompany him or her in this difficult part of the life journey.

LAW AND ETHICS

Law is a vital social structure. It enables people to live in community with some degree of security. However, law is neither primary nor exhaustive in ordering human affairs; neither is its objective to encourage virtue. Such functions are within the domain of ethics and morality, philosophy and religion. Law is necessary but often clumsy. Its sanctions are penalties and material incentives. Ethics and morality inform conscience; their sanction lies with the individual's and society's sense of right and wrong.

Moral agency is at the heart of humanness. It is rooted in our ability to form ideas and to order our actions in accord with these ideas (read "values" when ideas are applied to concrete decisions). To be a moral agent is to make judgments about the goodness of a proposed action, to choose a course of action and to hold oneself accountable, internally and externally, for the choice and its consequences.

The PSDA is a useful legal structure, but will have real meaning only if it furthers ethical behavior on the part of the potential patient, surrogate, family, significant others, and providers, both individual and institutional.

ETHICS: CARING AND CURING

Ethics is the systematic study of the appropriateness of human behavior. It addresses processes whereby human actions should be judged and specific situations about which human beings must make decisions. It is based on a perception of what it is to be human; in what human dignity consists; how society should function; and how humans should live within the context of the environment. Applied ethicists and ethical processes, such as ethics committees, attempt to help moral actors who are stakeholders in a given set of circumstances to make decisions and to take actions which are in accord with sound standards.

Even ethics can become quite sterile and reductionist if it emphasizes only process and decisionmaking without recognizing that its task is to forward decency for the individual, the person's social network, and society. Analogously, an advanced directive should not be viewed as a disembodied, technical instrument standing apart from the human journey. Medical decisions, whether they contribute to the restoration of health and functioning or are part of a dying process, are among the most critical moral choices a person can make. Indeed, to the degree in which they involve others, either as surrogates or as agents, they profoundly influence the moral character and psychological well being of others.

As important as appropriate decisions are, they are but part of the process in which human beings attend to one another in time of suffering. Ethical decisions contribute to, but do not exhaust, the curing and/or caring elements of health care.

THE MORAL LANDSCAPE

In the real world of caring and curing, it is important to identify the moral stakeholders and the nature of the human exchanges which occur. In the first instance, there is the person who is or may become a patient. There is the person who is chosen and agrees to be a surrogate. Then there are the persons who are the instrumental causes in implementing the wishes of the person. Often, treatment or nontreatment involves not one but many persons, each of whom becomes a moral stakeholder. Last but not least, there are the settings in which the decision(s) will be made or implemented.

Institutional Moral Responsibility

By analogy, institutions and agencies, to the degree that they are the creation of humans and have a corporate "life," also have the rights and responsibilities of legal and moral agents. Implicit and perhaps explicit in their behavior are convictions about the human condition. They are accountable for their acts or those carried out by their agents.

We are members of society. It has claims on us as we do on it. Its values, particularly as they find expression in regulation or in the ethos of the sponsor of the institution or agency, are also a factor in the moral calculus of decisionmaking.

In order to acquit their legal and moral responsibilities, the institution and agency must deal explicitly with both substantive and process matters which will be reflected in its policies, procedures, credentialing activities and in-service training. The institution or agency has a being which is both legal and moral. Implicitly and explicitly, it reflects the values of its "controlling persons" and the values which they choose to make explicit or to accept implicitly by reason of the behaviors which they allow, condone, or encourage in their moral domain.

The substantive issues should be decided within the context of each institution or agency's understanding of its vision, mission, rootedness, and values. There are, though, considerations common to all agencies and institutions, particularly as they involve themselves in the ethics of the interactions between its agents, i.e., those who provide service within its sponsorship and those who seek its services.

It may sound strange to speak of an institution's moral responsibility, but I think it appropriate. Institutions have a legal personality which involves rights and responsibilities. I would assert that it has a moral personality as well. One of the distinguishing characteristics of a health care agency is that it has a high moral purpose. The role of health care is to ameliorate the suffering of people: to heal and rehabilitate where possible, to support when such are not possible, and to help people to die well when that part of the human journey is imminent. What is more, we in the health care system recognize that our client is not merely the person who is sick, but also those people who are part of his or her life, who are affected by the patient's illness, and who in turn affect the patient.

Our agencies have their roots in communities that recognize that we are our brothers' and sisters' keeper. We are not dealing in a commodity but sharing in profoundly human dramas, including that of death.

As a moral being an institution should have a "philosophy" of life, embodied in values and reflective processes to measure its behavior in the light of its avowed goals and purposes. It professes a commitment to both paternalism (maternalism) and autonomy. It must use its capacity to help. It must empower the patient, not only physically and emotionally, but morally as well. In this role, the agency assists the patient to be an active participant in his or her life journey by assisting the patient to make informed decisions. The PSDA involves not only the discovery of an advance directive, but also serves as a teaching vehicle through which people can better understand both their rights and responsibilities.

The Patient

The ability to think and to act freely are marks of our humanness. The price of these qualities, unique to the human species, is responsibility. We must be moral agents not only in regard to others and the environment, but in regard to ourselves. This is true when it comes to health, whether in maintaining it or trying to restore it. We must be active agents and not merely passive spectators. Our tendency to procrastinate seems to be exacerbated when we are faced with actions which remind us of our mortality. Cemetery plots, wills, and now advance directives are readily put off for another day. In two studies done as part of the Retirement Research Foundation's Enhancing the Autonomy in Long Term Care Initiative, many older persons expressed the desire to delegate treatment decisions to their children or professional helpers (High, 1988; Wetle, Levkoff, Ciwikel, & Rosen, 1988).

Just, if not more, important than PSDA's primary function of supplying information to the agency so that it can follow the patient's wishes is its contribution to the patient's and the community's understanding of the importance of participating in treatment decisions. One of the elements in the changing health provider-patient relationship is a growing recognition that the patient must be an active participant in the therapeutic process if it is to be effective. Good practice and good ethics go hand in hand.

The Surrogate

In the instance of a health proxy or a durable power of attorney, the surrogate decisionmaker becomes an important figure, the one chosen to accompany the person in this

often difficult part of life. Surely, to be so chosen is a mark
of love and respect. To accept the designation involves the
same attributes. For the conscientious person, acting on behalf of another may be even more difficult than acting for
oneself. To fulfill the moral or ethical responsibilities inherent in such a designation, both designator and designee
should enter into a conversation so that both understand as
much as is humanly possible about how each feels, not only
about health care but about one another. Surely this is a
heavy responsibility on both parts. Additionally, it is important that significant others understand that such a designation has been made and why. It is vital that they accept the
person's wishes.

The Decisionmaking Field

Just as ethical decisions usually involve a conflict between or among two or more values and between or among
two or more persons, the moral field of decisionmaking is
often convoluted and complex. Usually, there is not one decision to be made, but many. Each has its own significance.
Each can involve different stakeholders. It is a trying and
confusing time for the competent patient and, in the instance of the incompetent person, for the surrogate
decisionmaker.

The stakeholders have differing roles, strengths, and vul-
nerabilities. While health care providers may be accus-
tomed to difficult decisions, patients and surrogates are
not. This milieu is strange and can be frightening for them.
Even elemental privacy can be lacking. The physical place
is filled with strange sights, sounds, and smells. Even the
language may be like something from another planet. The
providers are cloaked in professionalism and authority and
are not only familiar with, but in charge of, the environment. Most importantly, they are assumed to have knowledge about what is causing suffering here and now and how
it may be remedied.

While the decision or better decisions are critical in this

period and contribute to patient autonomy, neither they nor autonomy can assure dignity or peace. These goals require sensitivity, skill, caring and compassion on the part of all who are moral stakeholders.

CONCLUSION

The PSDA is another important step in society's attempts to catch up with technology. However, it is just a step. Fundamental questions about suffering, dependency, and death continue to intrude themselves in theory and in the instance of every person and dear one who experiences them. Our world, filled with new techniques and devices, continues to challenge philosophers, theologians, and legal experts, but most touchingly, frightened patients and those who love them and care for them. The PSDA can contribute to identifying moral agency, but such a contribution will not realize its full potential unless and until all involved recognize their rights and responsibilities both as moral agents and as caring human beings.

REFERENCES

High, D. M. (1988, June). All in the family: Extended autonomy and expectations in surrogate health care decision-making. *Gerontologist* 28 (Supplement): 46–51.
Wetle, T., Levkoff, S., Ciwikel, J., & Rosen, A. (1988, June). Nursing home resident participation in medical decisions: Perceptions and preferences. *Gerontologist* 28 (supplement): 32–38.

Self-Determination and Long-Term Care

2

William N. Kavesh, M.D., M.P.H.

The provisions of the Patient Self-Determination Act apply to a number of long-term care settings in which the physician ought to play a major role: home care, skilled nursing facilities, and nursing facilities for chronic care of the frail elderly. In many ways, the physician is the ideal person to help patients and family make difficult health care decisions, since most of these decisions affect care choices which physicians must authorize or carry out. In practice, however, things are not so simple. A review of the ambiguous role of the physician in long-term care may help to set matters straight.

Although the physician must, in fact, authorize all home medical, skilled, and chronic nursing facility services, policymakers have been concerned for decades about the limited physician presence in these settings (Kavesh, 1986). Data collected in the 1970s and 1980s indicate that few physicians make nursing home visits, and that those that do often did not represent the mainstream of American medicine (Mitchell, 1982). Speakers at two symposia held a decade ago, under the auspices of the American College of Physicians and National Foundation for Long Term Care, respectively (American College of Physicians, 1980; National Foundation for Long Term

11

Care, 1981) identified a myriad of concerns that discourage physician involvement, including excessive paperwork, inadequate reimbursement, and inappropriate attitudes about aging. Studies have shown that physician visits to nursing homes are often clustered in patterns that are driven by Medicare reimbursement intervals rather than obvious patient need (Willemain & Mark, 1980). As a result of these pressures, excessive nursing home care takes place in emergency situations, where physicians unfamiliar with the previously expressed wishes of a patient or family may make hasty decisions with major long-term consequences based upon limited information available at the time (Kavesh, Mark, & Kearney, 1984). Similar issues affect physician behavior in home care settings as well.

A number of changes have taken place in the past decade which have provided a certain optimism about the possibilities for expanding the physician's role in long-term care. Geriatrics has emerged on the American scene as a distinct specialty, with its own body of academic knowledge, research, and specialized expertise in areas such as cognitive dysfunction, gait disorders, incontinence, medication interactions, exercise physiology, osteoporosis, and functional assessment. Research into the illnesses affecting nursing home residents has expanded significantly, and the body of knowledge available to physicians practicing in nursing homes is now impressive (Ouslander, Osterweil, & Morley, 1991; Ouslander, 1989). Geriatric fellowships have developed at over 60 medical schools. The American Board of Internal Medicine and the American Academy of Family Practice jointly offer a biannual examination leading to a Certificate of Added Competence in Geriatrics, and specialty societies, such as the American Geriatrics Society and the American Academy of Home Care Physicians, have grown considerably in membership.

Under the nursing home reform provisions of the Omnibus Budget Reconciliation Act (OBRA) of 1987, all Medicare and Medicaid certified nursing facilities must now have a medical director who will oversee the quality of care provided by physician and nonphysician health care workers. The role of the nursing home physician has been expanded to include not only traditional medical care activities, but also participation in multidisciplinary assessments, determination of decision-making capacity, and a variety of other activities (Levenson, 1993). The American Medical Directors Association was formed to educate physicians who practice in nursing home settings and advocate for their interests. Physician reimbursement reform (the Resource Based Relative Value Scale, or RBRVS), mandated by the Omnibus Budget Reconciliation Act of 1990, promised to improve the financial incentives for such primary care activities as nursing home and home care visits.

It would appear, then, that the time was ripe for a major expansion of the role of the physician in long-term care. Unfortunately, the results have been more mixed. The RBRVS did improve reimbursements for home visits. It also improved reimbursement for hospital visits. But for providing evaluation and management services which are comparable to those in the hospital, the reimbursement for a nursing home visit will only reach hospital visit levels in 1996—hardly the incentive for an expansion of physician interest in nursing home care. Furthermore, despite all the financial tinkering under RBRVS, a physician choosing to practice gastroenterology can still expect to earn at least 50% more than a physician choosing a career in primary care ("Physician Earnings Survey," 1993).

Perhaps in response to these financial realities, there has been a major decline in the numbers of physicians entering primary care specialties such as general internal medicine and family practice, which is the major reservoir of physicians interested in geriatrics and primary care. According to the Association of American Medical Colleges, the number of 1992 medical school graduates indicating interest in specialty certification in general internal medicine was 1/3 of the number in 1985. The number showing an interest in family practice has undergone a decline of 30% over the same period (Kassebaum & Green, 1992). Conservative manpower estimates indicate that approximately 20,000 geriatricians are now needed to care for the over 30 million Americans over the age of 65. By 1992, only 4100 physicians had been certified as geriatricians (Alliance for Aging Research, 1992). Thus, for the foreseeable future, there is likely to be a shortage of physicians who have an interest in those nuances of the care of the elderly optimally required to assist patients and their families in making the often difficult choices among life-sustaining or rejecting treatment options.

Despite this mixed picture of incentives and disincentives for physicians to practice in long-term care settings, physicians who choose to devote a portion of their practice to long-term care often actively involve themselves in issues related to patient health care choices. The physician may be involved in numerous aspects of the decisionmaking process:

1) Assessment of decisionmaking capacity;
2) Explanation of the technical issues involved in various health care options;
3) Assessment of views of the patient;
4) Assessment of views of family members;
5) Consensus building among family members;
6) Interpretation of the decision to other health care providers at the nursing home or home care setting;
7) Interpretation of the decision to health care providers in the acute hospital setting;
8) Interactions with the designated surrogate; and
9) Reevaluation of options as the situation changes.

A review of the role of the physician in each of these areas, and the physician's role in safeguarding patient autonomy, will show the complexity of the issues involved.

AUTONOMY

The concept of personal autonomy underlies the process of all contemporary health care decisionmaking (American

Association of Retired Persons (AARP), 1992; President's Commission for the Study of Ethical Problems in Medicine and Biomedical and Behavioral Research, 1982). A person who is found to have decisionmaking capacity has the right to make all decisions regarding his/her health care, whether in the home, nursing home, or hospital. While this idea should perhaps be self-evident, in fact there are a number of complicating factors which affect physician decisionmaking in this area, especially in long-term care settings. First, most residents of nursing homes—63% of nursing home residents in 1985—are cognitively impaired (U.S. Senate Special Committee on Aging, 1991). This does not necessarily mean that they lack decisionmaking capacity (see below), but in many cases, this will be the case.

Second, even in situations where the person is not decisionally impaired, physicians sometimes find themselves under pressure by families to make decisions which reflect the psychological needs, financial interests, or other agendas of family members. Because the physician finds her/himself dealing so often with family members of impaired patients, it is easy to continue such arrangements even when dealing with decisionally capable patients, especially if the patient is hard of hearing, has other communication problems, speaks a different primary language, or is otherwise incapable of making him/herself easily understood. Furthermore, one should not underestimate the hassle factor in this area. Physicians are well aware that elderly patients rarely bring lawsuits and complaints to state medical boards or other agencies, but their children may.

Even without these formal threats, there are convenience factors that mitigate toward cooperation with interested parties. The nursing home administrator may want a resident sent to the hospital despite the resident's desire to remain at the nursing facility for care of an acute illness. In this case, the administrator may want to avoid the heavier care stress for staff, and the physician may find it more lucrative to care for the resident in the hospital. Families may pressure for hospital care as well, and the physician may decide that the risk of an adverse outcome at the nursing home, even if small, isn't worth it. Bucking family members can be a time-consuming task. The author is personally familiar with situations in which it appeared that a family member had a vested interest in a particular outcome and put pressure on at multiple levels to achieve that outcome.

CASE

A family member appears out of the woodwork from 3000 miles away to take over the care of his mother from a local friend and to push for her discharge from a nursing home. It soon becomes apparent that there may be financial issues at stake, since the resident is a private pay patient and apparently has a considerable sum of money. The physician questions whether the patient could function independently at home. The relative brings in a threatening lawyer and convinces the resident's friend, who has a power of attorney, that he was right. The resident has significant self-care deficits and borderline decisionmaking capacity. She keeps changing her mind as to what she wants to do. The nursing home administrator does not want a fight on his hands. Finally, after making detailed arrangements for home care followup and obtaining a "guarantee" that the patient will get daily visits from a neighbor, the physician agrees to discharge the patient.

CASE

A child of a patient pays detailed attention to all aspects of her nursing home care, and demands to be kept aware of both minor and major care changes. She questions the quality of the nursing home care frequently and insists that her father be given every possible intervention at the nursing home and at the hospital. The patient is not so sure that this is what he wants, but does not want to argue forcefully with his daughter. He has decisionmaking capacity. Restricting the daughter's visits or input does not seem feasible. The physician finds that the only way to deal with the situation is to have frequent conversations with the resident and play these back to the daughter, even when she later says that her father wants something else.

DETERMINATION OF DECISIONMAKING CAPACITY

Despite the prevalence of the concept of autonomy in contemporary medical decisionmaking, there is an equally widespread notion that the right to make health care choices may devolve onto someone else in certain circumstances. In the courts, this is defined as loss of competency, "the global ability to participate in the full range of daily transactions of society" (American Bar Association, 1991, p. 14). However, increasingly, health care institutions have chosen to make choices on the basis of decisional capacity, a concept articulated by the President's Commission for the Study of Ethical Problems in Medicine and Biomedical and Behavioral Research in 1982 (President's Commission, 1982). According to the President's Commission:

> Decisional capacity requires, to greater or lesser degree: (1) possession of a set of values and goals; (2) the ability to communicate and to understand information; and (3) the ability to reason and to deliberate about one's choices. (p. 57)

For the purposes of this chapter, we shall use the term "decisionmaking capacity" as synonymous with "decisional capacity."

In long-term care settings, the physician is often called upon to assess decisionmaking capacity. While the physician should have the ultimate responsibility for determining decisionmaking capacity (as opposed to legal competence), s/he will usually need to seek input from family and other staff, including, as appropriate, consultants from the fields of nursing, social work, psychology, and psychiatry. In some states, a second licensed practitioner (a psychologist or other professional) may also be required to participate in the determination (AARP, 1992).

Key attributes that a physician will want to assess include an understanding of information about the patient's current condition, treatment options, and the risk/benefit burden; judgment of this information in light of her/his values and goals; and the ability to communicate her/his decisions in a consistent and meaningful way. The fact that a person may not know the day of the week or be able to repeat a list of data may not prevent that person from understanding the implication of a particular treatment option.

Decisionmaking capacity also fluctuates from time to time. The physician must be attentive to the fact that intercurrent illness can produce temporary or permanent incapacity for decisionmaking. One should not automatically assume that the loss of decisionmaking capacity is permanent. Repeat examinations should be done as an illness improves.

Finally, all health care providers need to understand that our capability of discerning what a person knows and does not know is very primitive. Patients who do not pass standard tests of decisionmaking capacity still may be very much aware of what is going on around them and understand the implications of that activity even if they appear to forget what one tells them five minutes later.

CASE

An 85-year-old nursing home resident has become quite demented, although she can still play dominos with her daughter. Unexpectedly, her husband dies and her daughter comes to tell her. The old woman repeats, you mean he's gone to heaven?" The daughter says "Yes." The next day, she asks where her husband is and the daughter repeats the same story. This happens a few more times. Each time, the story seems to be new information. Shortly thereafter, she begins to eat poorly despite the efforts of her family to feed her. She loses weight and develops pneumonia. She seems to be getting better when she dies in her sleep.

Although there is no test to prove this, it seems unlikely to be simply a coincidence that this woman went downhill right after her husband died, even though she could not articulate her reactions. Nonverbal cues, such as spitting out food or pulling out tubes, are powerful guides to the thinking of demented patients who cannot express themselves in ways that meet the usual standards for decision-making capacity.

THE RANGE OF ISSUES FOR CONSIDERATION IN ADVANCE DIRECTIVES

It sometimes appears that the issues involved in health care decisionmaking really boil down to only two categories: well-publicized situations such as cardiac resuscitation, ventilator life-support, or feeding tubes; and everything else. In fact, as will be discussed in some detail below, the issues are far more general. As others indicate in this book, living wills generally apply to situations involving terminal illness, permanent vegetative state, or irreversible coma. Some state laws also specifically mention the withholding/withdrawal of nutrition and hydration.

However, most patient care situations involving options for withholding of treatment do not involve terminal illness. For example, there are very good reasons why most nursing home residents would want to choose to refuse resuscitation in the event of a cardiac arrest. Survival rates are abysmal. In one recently reported study, only 2 of 117 attempted resuscitations of nursing home residents were temporarily successful, and both residents died shortly thereafter (Applebaum, King, & Finucane, 1990). Other studies show similar results (Murphy, Murray, Robinson, & Campion, 1989). But, living wills describe only a limited spectrum of the situations likely to result in cardiac arrest. In fact, cessation of heart function most often occurs abruptly in the course of an acute heart or lung problem, and not simply as the final event of a terminal illness. Therefore, living wills have limited utility as a basis for doctor-patient discussion of the range of possible issues that should be addressed in an advanced directive.

In fact, although attention usually focuses on only a few well-publicized situations, the number of issues that one might consider for advanced directives in general is enormous. Furthermore, the complex details that must be mastered to understand any one of them and to assess the risk/ benefit ratio are often daunting even to sophisticated patients and their families. It may be useful, therefore to describe the technical aspects of some of the more common issues that confront patients and their families when considering an advance directive.

TECHNICAL ISSUES INVOLVED IN ADVANCED DIRECTIVES

The following are descriptions of the technical issues involved in advance directives. They are given so that the lay reader can get some idea of what patients and families must understand in order to make a decision about the various care options that are presented to them by their physicians.

Cardiopulmonary Resuscitation

When the heart stops, the lungs usually do as well, and it is therefore necessary to pay attention to both maintenance of breathing and heart pumping in resuscitation. The term "cardiopulmonary," which is often used by professionals, refers to cessation of heart (cardiac) and pulmonary (lung) function; the lay literature may often simply refer to "cardiac" resuscitation.

Since the first demonstration of successful cardiopulmonary resuscitation in 1963, physicians have discussed the possibility of resuscitation in the event of cardiac arrest with patients who seem at particular risk. Most physicians would not have such a discussion with a 40-year-old man having a hernia repair because they assume, probably correctly, that a 40-year-old otherwise healthy person would want to be resuscitated in the unlikely event that an arrest would occur. No such presumption can be made in the case of a nursing home resident or home care patient, who usually has multiple medical problems. Many geriatricians will now discuss the question of cardiopulmonary resuscitation with all nursing home or home care patients.

The specific issues involved in cardiopulmonary resuscitation of the elderly can usually be explained fairly straightforwardly. One of the key goals is to maintain the flow of oxygen into the patient's lungs. To do this, the physician, or another person trained in cardiopulmonary resuscitation, places a special bag over the patient's mouth. The bag pushes air in and allows it to flow out, like a bellows. When the bag is used, some of the air is invariably forced into the stomach. This happens because the esophagus, which carries food from the throat to the stomach, is also expanded by the air flowing into the mouth. If possible, a plastic tube is inserted through the nose or mouth and directed into the upper airways of the lungs. This is called *intubation*. The bag is then connected to the tube, allowing all the air from the bag to go directly to the lungs, rather than losing some into the stomach.

While air is being pushed in by the bag, blood circulation is maintained by external compression of the breast bone located in the middle of the chest. Since the heart is located below the breastbone, each compression flattens the heart and sends blood into the arteries. When the pressure is released, the heart expands, sucking new blood into it before the next compression. Medications to stimulate the heart may also be injected into the veins. This process is continued until the heart starts beating on its own or it becomes apparent that the process is futile.

Cardiopulmonary resuscitation, aside from being invariably unsuccessful in the nursing home setting, also has side effects. The most common aftermath is the pain from compression of the breastbone and adjacent ribs. Older people often have frail bones, and rib fractures are not uncommon after resuscitation attempts. After a period of *intubation*, the voice is hoarse and painful. While the tube is in the nose or mouth, it is impossible to talk, which can be quite frustrating. The air passed into the stomach instead of the lungs can cause painful swelling. Older patients who survive one episode of cardiac resuscitation have been known to admonish their physicians "never to do that again." Others may feel differently.

There is one circumstance in which cardiac arrest may be treated fairly successfully in all age groups. Patients undergoing surgery who develop a cardiac arrest during the procedure can often be successfully resuscitated. The higher success rate is probably due to the fact that the patient receiving general anesthesia for surgery is already intubated and the heart and lung function is being monitored second by second. Therefore, the problem is recognized and treated almost instantaneously. Physicians who discuss resuscitation with patients are often put in the difficult position of trying to explain how resuscitation can succeed in some circumstances but not others. Since some hospitals will not permit surgery to be done on a patient with a "do not resuscitate" order, it is best for physicians to anticipate such problems at the time of the initial discussion, rather than wait until a surgical emergency occurs in the middle of the night and then try to explain why the "do not resuscitate" order must be rescinded.

Ventilator Support

Support of respiratory function can be accomplished indefinitely by use of a machine which automatically pushes air into the lungs through a tube. Ventilators are used for patients whose lungs are too weak or damaged to expand enough to draw air into them, who have fluid in the walls of the lung tissue that blocks the exchange of gases, or whose brain function is damaged so that automatic control of respirations is lost. In principle, the process is the same as the use of the bag and tube above, except that the machine replaces the person squeezing the bag. After a period of a week or two, the pressure of a tube in the lung airways can cause damage and it is usually replaced with a tracheostomy tube, a shorter tube inserted through an incision in the lower neck. Tracheostomy tubes can be maintained or changed much more easily than tubes placed through the nose or mouth and they are more comfortable. As noted above, it is impossible to talk while a tube is connected to a ventilator.

A person being treated with a ventilator who is awake enough to perceive what is happening often finds it very uncomfortable. Discomfort may occur because the ventilator has been set to deliver respirations at a certain level to maintain a proper balance of oxygen and other body gases, while the person wants to breathe either faster or less deeply. This is sometimes called "fighting the respirator." In these circumstances, the physician may use medications to cause the person to relax. In unusual circumstances, the physician may even use medications to paralyze the muscles so that the respirator can do its work unopposed. This produces loss of control of all muscles in the body, which may be an upsetting experience.

Feeding Tubes

Swallowing is a complex mechanism involving the synergistic action of the tongue, muscles of the front and back of the mouth, muscles of the throat, and, finally, the esophagus, the tube which carries food from the lower throat to the stomach. A key to successful swallowing is muscular coordination of all these functions, together with proper closing of a muscular cap to the windpipe, which prevents food from going into the lungs. One of the common problems interfering with swallowing is a stroke, which may interfere with the ability to move food from the front to the back of the mouth and into the esophagus. A stroke may also prevent the proper coordination of swallowing so that food may inadvertently enter the lungs and cause pneumonia.

A second common problem, especially affecting nursing home residents, is the inability to swallow properly due to dementia. Regardless of the cause, whether it is Alzheimer's Disease or another type, many patients with advanced dementias lose the ability to coordinate swallowing just as they lose the ability to perform other coordinated activities. The result is the same as a swallowing problem due to a stroke. The other problem affecting patients with dementia is simply loss of the capacity, or capability, for taking in food. Many patients with advanced dementias will take only tiny amounts of food or liquid at a time. It may take 2 to 3 hours to feed such a person the equivalent of a single meal. A syringe may have to be used to place food into the person's mouth.

Feeding tubes are used in situations where a person is unable to swallow without allowing some of the food to enter the lungs or is unable or unwilling to take food into her/his mouth. Feeding tubes fall into two categories: those inserted through the nose down the back of the throat and esophagus to the stomach, and those which extend through the abdominal wall directly into the stomach. The first type of feeding tube, called a *nasogastric* tube, must be placed by the physician through the nose and throat. If the patient can cooperate, s/he is usually encouraged to swallow a small amount of water through a straw to draw the tube from the throat into the stomach. The tube does not always go down the first time. Sometimes, it can inadvertently go down the windpipe to the lung. Usually, but not always, the physician is alerted to this because the patient coughs. Sometimes, it is only noticed when a chest x-ray is obtained after the tube is placed to see that it is in proper position. Patients often find a nasogastric feeding tube uncomfortable at first and will yank it out if given the opportunity. Therefore, they are sometimes restrained.

The second type of feeding tube is one which extends directly through the abdominal wall into the stomach, sometimes called a *PEG* tube because of the name of the procedure most commonly used to put it in: percutaneous endoscopic gastrostomy. At one time, these tubes were put in by a surgical procedure from outside to inside. Currently, they are usually placed from inside to outside via the use of an endoscope, an instrument about the thickness of an office telephone wire which reaches into the stomach and through which the inside of the stomach can be visualized. Instruments for cutting can also be passed through the endoscope.

In order to pass an endoscope, the patient's throat is sprayed with a Novocaine-like anesthetic to prevent gagging and a sedative is given intravenously. Then the endoscope is passed down the throat into the stomach. Through the endoscope, a tiny cut is made in the wall of the stomach and then through the subsequent walls of the abdomen. Then the feeding tube is passed out to the surface and a balloon is blown up to hold it inside the stomach. The patient usually is quite drowsy throughout the endoscopy. Nondemented patients describe the procedure as mildly uncomfortable. Once in place, a PEG tube is often tolerated better than a nasogastric tube. After some time passes, most patients seem to become relatively unaware of its presence.

Once a tube is in place, specially formulated liquid feedings are pumped down the tube by a portable pump which draws the feeding from a bag held on a pole at the side of the bed. While the pump is running, the patient must be kept in a sitting position in the bed to avoid regurgitating and aspirating the feeding, possibly causing pneumonia—the condition which insertion of the tube is sometimes supposed to prevent in the first place.

Everything Else

While the classic triad of resuscitation, ventilation, and feeding tubes usually come to mind as the subject of advance directives, in fact, there are a number of other medical conditions which may affect a person's attitude toward the intensity or type of treatments which that person may desire.

For example, arthritis may produce chronic pain that limits movement and requires the use of medications several times a day. The medications may cause stomach upset, nausea or constipation, and may not fully control the pain. As a result, the overall quality of that person's life may deteriorate.

Severe heart problems may also affect a person's attitudes and choices. Congestive heart failure is a condition caused by inability of the heart to pump the blood adequately through the body. Because of this weakness, fluid backs up into the lungs and the legs. The fluid in the lungs prevents the body from getting adequate oxygen for its normal functions, often producing shortness of breath on the slightest activity or generalized fatigue. The person can have acute attacks of air hunger at night. Frequent adjustments of medication may be necessary plus blood tests as often as several times a week to monitor the effects of medication changes.

Similarly, impairment of brain function may change a person's perception of the quality of her life. A person who had formerly been independent may suddenly have a stroke that leaves her with weakness on one side of her body and the inability to talk or understand the speech of others. This eliminates her favorite activity: walking around to different floors of the nursing home and visiting her friends. Another common scenario which can have profound implications is one in which a person may begin to notice a progressive loss of memory and ability to keep track of conversations, possibly an early sign of dementia.

These and other chronic debilitating illnesses may prompt a person to reevaluate his or her life goals and decisionmaking about the extent of treatment desired for the primary illness or for intercurrent illnesses. The role of the physician in these situations is to explain what the likely course of the chronic illness may be; how the effects of an acute illness may interact with the chronic illness; and what would happen if the person were to choose options ranging from care designed to maximize comfort to the maximum treatment possible.

ASSESSMENT OF THE VIEWS OF THE PATIENT

The goal of the physician in discussing advance directives should be to present whatever information is necessary for the patient to advise the physician, family members, or other surrogates of his/her general values and specific wishes in the event that the patient is no longer able to make personal decisions. One of the major problems associated with living wills and other advance directive documents is that they provide only a limited amount of guidance for a few specific situations (Lynn, 1991). A more versatile approach is to ascertain not only a person's views about specific situations, but their general set of values, which may guide others who may need to make decisions when the person becomes incapacitated. For example, some value areas which a person might consider in advising a surrogate or health provider are set out in the advance directive document used at the Philadelphia Geriatric Center (see Appendix, "Instructions to my Surrogate," for text of the full document). These values include the desire to live as long as possible, even if the ability to function becomes impaired; to maintain dignity; to have a satisfying quality of life; to be able to communicate with other people; and to be free from pain. The resident has the opportunity to elaborate on each of these to whatever degree s/he wishes.

Following the values section of the Philadelphia Geriatric Center document is a section which allows the resident to describe his/her wishes regarding approaches to treatment in the event that his/her chronic illness becomes progressively more life-threatening, if an acute illness supervenes in addition to the chronic illness, or if the resident develops cognitive impairment. The choices available are presented as a Likert scale continuum from comfort care only to maximum treatment. Finally, a list of specific treatments is given with a set of three or four options for each. The physician will need to explain these to the patient and attempt to elicit as accurately as possible what the patient's true wishes are.

A major issue for physicians in this situation is to ascertain what the resident truly wants, as opposed to what the family may want or what the physician's underlying values may dictate. A considerable literature has arisen in the past few years suggesting that there is sometimes a poor correlation between what patients say they want and what their physicians think they want. In one study (Uhlmann & Pearlman, 1991), primary physicians rated the global quality of life of their older, chronically ill patients as being significantly worse than did the patients themselves. The physicians' more negative perceptions of their patients' quality of life also colored the physicians' attitudes toward life sustaining treatment for these patients. On the other hand, the patients showed little correlation between most quality of life dimensions and their preferences for life-sustaining treatment.

Other studies have also shown poor congruence between the predictions of physicians and close relatives and the actual resuscitation preferences indicated by the patients (Uhlmann, Pearlman, & Cain, 1988; Ouslander, Tymchuk, & Rahbar, 1989). Thus, physicians assisting older patients in developing advance directives need to be particularly sensitive to listening, rather than permitting their own preconceptions to intrude.

On the other hand, there still are patients who prefer to delegate such decisions to others; in that circumstance, rigid insistence that all patients be required to exercise their rights to autonomy by making their own decisions can be just as oppressive as a thoroughgoing medical paternalism.

CASE

A 95-year-old perfectly alert matriarch of a distinguished family, attended by a number of physicians was asked to indicate her preferences regarding resuscitation in the event of a cardiac arrest. Her reply: "Let the doctors decide. They know best."

As noted earlier, about two-thirds of nursing home residents have cognitive impairment. This does not automatically mean that they are decisionally incapable. Furthermore, whereas a judge's determination of competency usually is a global judgment of a person's capacities (despite a recent recognition of the idea of limited or partial competence), and is not likely to be changed from time to time, decisionmaking capacity may vary from situation to situation. Many patients who cannot articulate their understanding of the risks and benefits of a complex surgical procedure can still be very clear that they do not want a leg amputated. As noted above, many of the situations that confront patients are not ones they thought about or for which they wrote guidelines. But, as a physician, one must take very seriously the opinion of a patient who says s/he does not want something done, even if the person is only marginally capable according to traditional criteria. Do no harm.

ASSESSMENT OF THE VIEWS OF FAMILY MEMBERS

Family members, by virtue of their close association with the nursing home resident or home care patient, are presumably in the best position to ascertain what that person's views would be in the event that s/he becomes unable to express her/his own views. As noted above, studies based on presentation of the same advance directive scenario to both patients and their families show that family members do not always guess so well what their relative would want. Nonetheless, they are likely to have the best understanding under the circumstances, since they are most likely to have a long-term sense of the patient's values and preferences.

The physician will usually find it prudent to talk to family members, both in situations where the patient has decision-making capacity and in situations where the patient does not.

Patients Without Decisionmaking Capacity

In nursing home settings, as noted earlier, almost two-thirds of residents are cognitively impaired. Although this does not automatically disqualify such a resident from having decisionmaking capacity, in many cases this will indeed be the case. If the resident has a durable power of attorney for health care or has otherwise left written instructions appointing a surrogate before or at the time of admission to the nursing home, the physician has a clear mandate to obtain permission from the appropriate person before making care decisions. This should certainly be done when the physician is attempting to obtain an advance directive for a contemplated problem about which the patient left no specific written instructions. But it also should be done in situations where the patient left specific instructions in order to be sure that the surrogate understands the instructions in the same way that the physician does.

In situations where a resident may not be capable of decisionmaking at the time of admission to a nursing home, a situation affecting a substantial proportion of new residents, nursing homes will often formally or informally deal with the family member who arranged the admission or with whom the elder had previously been living. The Philadelphia Geriatric Center currently has a policy of requesting that this person sign a paper agreeing to serve as a surrogate. This person is then asked to notify other family members to obtain their verbal assent to this arrangement. Administrative staff, not the physician, obtain these permissions and may even attempt to mediate with families if any members disagree about the appointment of surrogate.

Strictly speaking, the Patient Self-Determination Act deals only with the rights of patients who are decisionmakers. However, since the majority of nursing home residents have dementias and do not have advance directives on admission, a few words ought to be added about the physician's role in relation to surrogates who need to make decisions for their relatives. The task of the surrogate is not an easy one. The decision to shut off treatment for a parent or other relative is fraught with feelings of guilt and loss. I have found that, despite the tenor of the times, a physician may well be in the situation of advocating a particular position which s/he may know the patient would have wanted and which the surrogate is comfortable with—usually the withholding of treatment.

CASE

A 90-year-old gregarious woman who was prone to intermittent sadness, but who got great pleasure from walking about the nursing home and talking to other residents, suffered a stroke that paralyzed one side of the body and left her unable to understand conversation or to speak. She also had difficulty swallowing. When the physician came in to visit, she would raise her good arm and wave her hand in a sign of disgust. After 10 days of intravenous therapy, she was no better. She began to spit out the little food that she could get into her mouth. Her son was asked if a feeding tube should be placed. He clearly indicated to the physician that he had enormous difficulty making that decision, even though he felt that his mother's major pleasure was walking and talking to people. The physician initially suggested showing the feeding tube to the patient and seeing her reactions, but it became apparent that the patient could not understand what was being presented as an option. The physician knew from previous discussion with the patient that she had wanted to limit his therapeutic interventions in the event of a cardiac arrest so that she would not have a long period of life support. Realizing that the son felt too guilty to take the responsibility himself, the physician told the son that, based on everything he knew about the patient, he doubted that the patient would have wanted a feeding tube. The son agreed to withhold a feeding tube. The physician explained the decision to the nursing home staff who felt comfortable with the reasoning. Everyone agreed that the nursing staff would offer small amounts of food as tolerated by the patient. She died 3 days later.

Other Family Members

The prudent physician will be aware that the existence of an advance directive known to one family member or appointment of that person as a surrogate does not mean that other family members may not have a strong interest in understanding the medical condition of a parent or other relative. It is usually wise, at the time an advance directive is made, to explain it to all interested parties, so the physician has a clear idea what their views are and can answer any questions. If there are disagreements among family members about the implications of an advance directive, the physician should attempt to obtain consensus, so that these disagreements do not simply resurface when a decision actually has to be implemented.

On rare occasions, consensus can be very hard to achieve. Family members may have longstanding philosophical or personal disagreements and, in rare instances, may not even be willing to sit in the same room together. Although the process can be laborious and time-consuming—and may even involve talking to family members separately at times—it has been my experience that the conscientious physician can usually help family members to reach some type of understanding about what should happen in a given situation.

Patients With Decisionmaking Capacity

Physicians also need to talk to families in situations where advance directives have been made by patients who in fact are perfectly capable of making their own decisions. Family members have their own views and psychological needs, which may color their ability to support the advance directives of a patient who has decisionmaking capacity. A child may be unable to accept the possibility that a parent may die as a result of a decision made by the parent, even if it is clear that the parent has carefully thought through the consequences of her/his choice. Children can pressure parents to make choices which the parent tells others s/he does not really want. The role of the physician is to support the patient in making the decision which the patient wants.

At times, supporting the patient may put the physician in the position of confronting an angry relative who may deal with his/her anxieties by projecting his/her anger onto the physician, the institution, or others. The physician can minimize adverse consequences in such a situation by taking several measures.

First, document in detail any conversations with the patient which relate to the advance directive. Bring in other witnesses to a conversation with the patient. Do the same thing with conversations with the relative. If the relative is particularly recalcitrant, the state nursing home ombudsman, whose role is to advocate for the resident, can often be helpful and support the physician in his/her role as a patient advocate. If a problem reaches this stage, the physician should also notify the nursing home administrator of the issues and coordinate responses.

ASSESSMENT OF VIEWS OF HOME CARE PATIENTS AND THEIR FAMILIES

The issues in home care regarding advance directives are similar in a number of ways to the issues in institutional long-term care settings, but there are some unique features germane to the home care setting. Although the degree of dementia among patients served by home health agencies is only about 25%, compared to 63% noted earlier for nursing home patients (Marion Merrell Dow, 1993), the physician

will still be in the position of needing to determine decisionmaking capacity for these patients. In this situation,
the resources to support the physician may be more limited. If the patient needs neuropsychological testing to help
define decisional capacity in a borderline situation, the
physician will need to find a psychologist who makes house
calls.

On the other hand, the family decisionmaking hierarchy
is often clearer in the home setting. It is usually the family
member with whom the elder is living who takes prime responsibility for decisionmaking when the patient is incapable of doing so, and most other family members usually accept this. In the course of making home visits, the physician
usually develops a close working relationship with this per-
son/family unit because the person is providing a lot of personal care for the patient, even when there is professional
support from home health aides and others (Kavesh, 1986).
Only rarely will conflicts of interest arise with the primary
support person. When they do, the problems can be much
more difficult than those that arise in the nursing home, because both the patient and physician are depending on this
person to provide primary supportive care at home.

INTERPRETATION OF THE DECISION TO OTHER NURSING HOME OR HOME HEALTH CARE PROVIDERS

The physician's role in a long-term care setting is not limited simply to determining what the patient or family want
and then documenting the result. In both the nursing home
and home care settings, numerous staff establish relationships with patients over time. They can become a second
family for some patients. It should not be surprising, then,
that staff who do not understand why a particular decision
was made can be frustrated and upset at having to carry it
out. This is especially difficult in cases involving the use of
feeding tubes, for example, or terminal care of a patient

who has developed gangrene and refuses an amputation. The physician should talk to the nurses and nurses' aides who care for the patient and explain how the patient and/or the surrogate came to their decision. This is also an important time for the physician to find out the feelings of staff about the particular decision and what issues they might have in being supportive.

Usually the concerns are easily dealt with. Nurses and nurses' aides often want permission to offer food to a patient who has refused a feeding tube even when everyone knows that the patient will not get adequate nutrition and hydration, may aspirate, or may even refuse to eat most of the time. Staff caring for a patient with gangrene or other slowly terminal condition may need to know that the physician recognizes that it is hard for them to see someone die knowing that something might be done. They may suggest various options for care that they feel will make the patient (and themselves) more comfortable. In those circumstances, it is good for the physician to be flexible in the plan of care, consistent with the primary goal of providing maximum comfort to the patient. It is sometimes helpful to remind staff that the patient will be much more comfortable among those who know her/him in the nursing home or at home than being taken to a hospital with unfamiliar staff and surroundings.

INTERPRETATION OF THE DECISION TO HEALTH CARE PROVIDERS IN THE HOSPITAL

The physician who knows the patient's wishes in the long-term care setting plays an important role as an advocate for the patient in the acute hospital. Hospitals have a totally different ambiance than nursing homes. They are short-stay institutions whose focus is on diagnosis and cure, not long-term supportive care. The hospital environment does not encourage the withdrawal of care. A recent survey of physicians and nurses revealed the disturbing fact that almost half of them reported that they had acted against their conscience in providing care which simply prolonged the lives of terminally ill hospitalized patients, even though the doctors and nurses expressed general agreement with the right of dying patients to decline life-sustaining treatments. Furthermore, only one-third of those surveyed were satisfied that staff make the effort to find out what critically and terminally ill patients want (Solomon et al., 1993). The author of an editorial accompanying this report (Dubler, 1993) tries to reconcile these apparent contradictions by suggesting that "Beliefs . . . are not behavior" and that institutions may create a certain kind of moral inertia that frustrates providers who may want to behave in ways consonant with what they suspect their patients want (Dubler, 1993). This inertia seems to especially affect house staff, 70% of whom said they acted against their conscience, far more than medical attending physicians, only 38% of whom felt this way. House staff presumably are more influenced by what they feel the institutional environment dictates. Advance directives will not help solve this problem Attending physicians who are aware of their patients' advance directives will need to be vigilant to see that they actually are carried out.

The other problem that unfortunately can happen to patients who come from a long term care setting to the hospital is that the hospital will not recognize the advance directive obtained outside the hospital and will insist on talking to the patient or whatever family members they can find at the time. This sitaution highlights a major problem with advance directives. On the one hand, the whole point of making an advance directive is to permit the individual or surrogate to think through the issues in advance with someone they trust to provide them with appropriate information and guidance. On the other hand, people can change their minds. A person with decisionmaking capacity theoretically could decide that s/he wants to be intubated because she is short of breath. This scenario raises numerous problems. Many people with decisionmaking capacity at the time they make an advance directive may become confused during the course of an acute illness. An emergency room physician who does not know the patient is not likely to call for a neuropsychological consultant at 3 A.M. but rather will make an assessment of decisionmaking capacity based on the exigencies of the moment. The patient who passes this test may then be subjected to a variety of interventions that s/he had explicitly requested be withheld at the time the advance directive was executed.

If the person fails this test of decisionmaking capacity, whatever family member can be reached on the phone at that hour, even one who may have had ambivalent feelings about his/her relative's initial choice to limit interventions, may then opt for more aggressive treatment. The entire process may play itself out before the primary physician is ever contacted. Hospital lawyers who do not want the hospital to be faulted for inadequately treating the patient can contribute to this mindset (Dubler, 1993). Physicians need to work to establish emergency room protocols at their hospitals which will insure that the advance directives of their long-term care patients are not overturned in ambiguous situations.

The other side of the coin in acute care is the need to encourage appropriate intensive care for patients who need it even if they choose not to be resuscitated in the event of a cardiac arrest. I have personally experienced or heard from other physicians of situations where house staff feel that a patient who has a DNR status should not be permitted to receive intensive care. Hospitals have in some cases established policies to exclude such patients from the intensive care unit. The physician must advocate for the patient in these situations as well.

The patient who requires surgery is a special case. As noted earlier, if a patient closely monitored under anesthesia develops an arrhythmia which might be potentially fatal in an unmonitored setting, immediate treatment with medication or defibrillation may be life-saving. Therefore, it seems reasonable to limit DNR orders to settings outside

the operating room. The physician should try to explain the
possibility of this type of situation at the time the advance
directive is signed. But s/he may also need to remind the patient and surrogate at the time of potential surgery that the
DNR order will not apply to the operating room.

PERIODIC REVIEW OF THE ADVANCE DIRECTIVE

The physician should review the advance directive with the
patient or surrogate as often as necessary but at least once a
year. The patient or surrogate may have had some intervening
experience which colors her/his thinking in a new way and issues may have arisen with other family members.

The review should be very low-key. Anecdotal evidence
exists that, after agonizing to make the original decision,
especially a decision not to resuscitate or otherwise to
withhold therapy, surrogates can feel quite put upon when
asked to reopen the whole issue. The physician can be helpful in this regard by suggesting that he is simply notifying
the family about the option for an annual review or to discuss any new issues that might have arisen. If the patient
undergoes a major change in condition, of course, a more
complete discussion may be necessary.

As problems unfold that may result in activation of an
advance directive, the physician will usually find it helpful
to keep in touch with the designated surrogate. Many of the
scenarios do not unfold the way people envision them when
an advance directive is written. Good communication can
help everyone concerned.

CAVEATS AND CONCLUSIONS

In the past decade, the concept of autonomy has become
a major principle motivating decisionmaking activities in
the health care system. The Patient Self-Determination Act,
whose goal is to promote widespread knowledge of advance

directives (McCloskey, 1991), clearly follows in the spirit of this principle. However, there are a number of questions which will need to be addressed to determine how successful the PSDA ultimately will be in long-term care settings.

1) *How useful will the PSDA be if facilities simply hand out a piece of paper to prove to regulators that they have informed patients of their rights?* This response is, in fact, the one which harried hospital or long-term care administrators may find easiest to employ, and one which I have already seen at the hospital level. It is time-consuming for physicians to do the background work to help a patient and family decide on an advance directive. While a primary care physician may have had such discussions in the nursing home, under a hospital prospective payment system little incentive exists for hospital-based physicians, who may be meeting the patient for the first time, to undertake such time-consuming activities. Since some nursing home-based physicians do not follow their patients in the hospital, this can be a problem.

2) *How successful can PSDA be in nursing homes?* PSDA only applies to patients who are capable of making their own decisions. Most nursing home residents do not fall into this category. Nonetheless, because PSDA follows in the wake of the regulatory reforms spawned by the Omnibus Budget Reconciliation Act (OBRA) of 1987, especially those reforms dealing with residents' rights, compliance with the spirit of PSDA is likely to spill over into a general concern for maximizing the input of surrogates and somewhat impaired residents into their care plans.

3) *How successful are advance directives in affecting medical outcomes?* A 1985 study of the impact of a state Durable Power of Attorney for Healthcare, including placing a summary in the patient's chart, revealed "no significant positive or negative effect on patient's well being, health status, medical treatments, or medical treatment charges" (Schneiderman & Arras, 1985). Preliminary findings from a hospital-based study (the SUPPORT study) of

decisions in intensive care unit settings suggest that advance directives have only a small effect on the decision to choose cardiopulmonary resuscitation (Phillips, personal communication). However, this study included all age groups and did not have a particular focus on long-term care settings, where the nature of chronic illness and regulatory imperatives like OBRA '87 may stimulate greater awareness and provide the time to generate responses that remain relatively consistent. Only studies focused on the long-term care setting will help to tease out the impact of advance directives on nursing homes and home care.

4) *Are written instructions such as living wills sufficient?* Written instructions can never cover the range of nuances which invariably arise in a particular situation (Lynn, 1991). Physicians need to be able to discuss these issues with interested family or other surrogates in order to maximize the possibility that the outcome approximates what the patient would have wanted as closely as possible.

5) *Is the physician the only one who can talk with a patient or family members about PSDA?* The law is specifically vague about who can do this. Social workers, case managers, nurses, and other health professionals often have long term, trusting relationships with patients, and understand the nuances of their needs and fears. It is very appropriate for these health professionals to talk to patients and families about PSDA, obtain signatures regarding power of attorney or other designations of surrogates, and engage in general discussions of the issues around specific types of advance directive. However, as suggested above in the discussions of technical issues, decisions about specific matters can be complex, involving an assessment of current health status as well as the nature of the contemplated procedures. Medically skilled providers, such as advanced-practice nurses and physician assistants, can be very helpful in this area, but in most nursing home and home care settings this will usually be an appropriate area for the physician.

REFERENCES

Alliance for Aging Research. (1992). *Meeting the medical needs of the senior boom: The national shortage of geriatricians.* Washington, DC: Alliance for Aging Research.

American Association of Retired Persons. (1992). *A matter of choice: Planning ahead for health care decisions.* Washington, DC: American Association of Retired Persons.

American Bar Association. (1991). *Patient Self-Determination Act State Law Guide.* Washington, DC: Author.

American College of Physicians. (1980, June 12–13). *The changing needs of nursing home care.* Proceedings of the American College of Physicians Conference. Washington, DC: Author.

Applebaum, G. E., King, J. E., & Finucane, T. E. (1990). The outcome of CPR initiated in nursing homes. *Journal of the American Geriatric Society, 38,* 197–200.

Dubler, N. N. (1993). Commentary: Balancing life and death: Proceed with caution. *American Journal of Public Health, 83,* 23–25.

Kassebaum, D. G., & Green, D. (1992). Interest in generalist careers continues to wane. *Academic Physician, 10,* 4–5.

Kavesh, W. N. (1986). Home care: Process, outcome, cost. *Annual Review of Gerontology and Geriatrics, 6,* 135–195.

Kavesh, W., Mark, R., & Kearney, B. (1984, November). *Medical care teams improve nursing home care and reduce costs.* Paper presented at the 37th annual scientific meeting of the Gerontological Society of America, San Antonio, TX.

Levenson, S. A. (1993). *Medical direction in long-term care: A guidebook for the future* (2nd ed.). Durham, NC: Carolina Academic Press.

Lynn, J. (1991). Why I don't have a living will. *Law, Medicine, and Health Care, 19,* 101–104.

Marion Merrell Dow. (1993). *Managed care digest: Long-term care edition.* Kansas City, MO: Author.

McCloskey, E. L. (1991). The spirit of the PSDA. *Hastings Center Report, 21* 14–15.

Mitchell, J. B. (1982). Physicians' visits in nursing homes. *Gerontologist, 22,* 45–49.

Murphy, D. J., et al. (1989). Outcomes of cardiopulmonary arrest in the elderly. *Annals of Internal Medicine, 111,* 199–205.

National Foundation for Long-Term Care. (1981, May 23–24). Physician involvement in nursing homes. Proceedings of a conference. Washington, DC: Author.

Ouslander, J. G. (1989). Medical care in the nursing home. *JAMA*, *262*, 2582–90.

Ouslander, J. G., Osterweil, D., & Morley, J. (1991). *Medical care in the nursing home*. New York: McGraw-Hill.

Ouslander, J. G., Tymchuk, A. J., & Rahbar, B. (1989). Health care decisions among elderly long-term care residents and their potential proxies. *Gerontologist*, *29*, 615–21.

Physician earnings survey. (1993). *Medical Economics*, *70*, 101–112.

President's Commission for the Study of Ethical Problems in Medicine and Biomedical and Behavioral Research. *Making health care decisions*. (1982). Washington, DC: U.S. Government Printing Office.

Schneiderman, L. J., & Arras, J. D. (1985). Counseling patients to counsel physicians on future care in the event of patient incompetence. *Annals of Internal Medicine*, *102*, 693–98.

Solomon, M. Z., O'Donnell, L., Jennings, B., Guilfoy, V., Wolf W. M., Nolan, K., Jackson, R., Koch-Weser, D., & Donnelly, J. (1993). Decisions near the end of life: Professional views on life sustaining treatments. *American Journal of Public Health*, *83*, 14–22.

Uhlmann, R. G., & Pearlman, R. A. (1991). Perceived quality of life and preference for life-sustaining treatment in older adults. *Archives of Internal Medicine*, *151*, 495–97.

Uhlmann, R. F., Pearlman, R. A., & Cain, K. C. (1988). Physicians' and spouses' predictions of elderly patients' resuscitation preferences. *Journal of Gerontology*, *43*, M115–M121.

U.S. Senate Special Committee on Aging. (1991). *Aging America*. Washington, DC: Author.

Willemain, T. R., & Mark, R. G. (1980). The distribution of intervals between visits as a basis for assessing and regulation of physician services in nursing homes. *Medical Care*, *18*, 427–441.

Establishing an Ethics Committee for a Nursing Home

3

Todd L. Sobol, M.D., and
Sister Agnes Marie Boes, R.S.M.,
M.S.N., M.S.A.

ESTABLISHING PURPOSE AND OBJECTIVES

An institutional medical ethics committee may be established to insure the highest quality of patient care consistent with the mission of the institution and the rights of the individual patient. Establishment of policies and procedures for the long-term care facility will avoid most conflicts. However, due to the increasing complexities of medical care, the facility needs to have a means in place for arbitration. An ethics committee is in place to ensure a compassionate response to dilemmas of patients, family members, and staff.

The purpose of the ethics committee should not be to act as a decisionmaking entity. Proper functions may include: advising patients, families, physicians, and staff; facilitating communication; mediating between ethical theory and concrete medical judgments; providing support for those involved in painful decisions; assisting in policy formation;

providing education; and minimizing the institution's vulnerability to litigation (Drane & Roth, 1985).

COMMUNICATION

Good communication between all parties involved is a key to early and acceptable resolution of conflicts prior to arbitration. All parties should understand the medical and ethical options as clearly as possible. A "pyramid" of relationships illustrates where the ethics committee fits into the working relationship of patient care.

The relationship between the patient and personal physician sits atop the "pyramid." This relationship is influenced by the degree of physical and mental impairment of the patient, beliefs and values held by both individuals, and projected outcomes from treatment.

The next level deals with those who directly care for the patient. Family members may be influenced by the same issues as patients as well as by financial concerns and emotional issues. In the case of the terminally ill patient, for example, assisting family members to work through the grieving process along with their loved ones will be beneficial. Communication among multiple family members is a key factor in determining mutual agreement on a course of action. This task can place staff in the middle of established family conflicts.

Open lines of communication between the physician and the rest of the health care team allow clear explanation of directives. The free exchange of ideas and emotions allows all involved to reach a mutual understanding. Rules and regulations may constrain staff. The individual level of training and experience underscores the need for continuing education of health care workers.

The bottom levels are comprised of the support structure. The ethics committee is central to resolving dilemmas. The structure of this committee will be discussed below.

LEGAL ISSUES

Certain basic legal principles must be upheld when developing the ethics committee. The health care facility is responsible and liable for the quality of care rendered within it. This responsibility rests ultimately with the facility's governing board, which must ensure that sufficient policies and procedures are in place to optimize patient care. An ethics committee may serve as one mechanism to assure the accomplishment of this duty. In some states an ethics committee is legally mandated in some situations; e.g., New Jersey facilities following the *Quinlan* decision require a prognosis body; Maryland hospital ethics committees are required by statute.

The patient's right to privacy must be upheld. Information communicated within the doctor-patient relationship is privileged and confidential. Persons not directly involved in the patient's care must have the patient's permission to become privy to information that is identifiable as relating to the patient. This can be accomplished through a "consent form" signed by an authorized party, either on admission to the facility or at the time a conflict is brought forth.

Specific treatment decisions remain the physician's responsibility, in conjunction with the patient's informed consent. Therefore, the ethics committee's role is advisory and consultative rather than decisional. The physician may be discharged from the patient's care by the patient or authorized surrogates, or preempted by court order, provided another attending physician is in place.

There should be little danger of personal liability to committee members, provided the ethics committee functions in good faith. The facility may want to extend liability insurance coverage to its committee members. It can be assumed that any record of ethics committee activities will be discoverable and admissible in litigation. Therefore, minutes and other documents should be prepared and reviewed with accuracy and fairness in mind. The institution's legal counsel should be consulted for specific legal advice and questions regarding state laws.

DEVELOPING A PROTOCOL FOR THE COMMITTEE

Developing a protocol is like developing a road map for the committee. Instead of locating cities and towns, specific decision points are referenced. Another way of thinking about a protocol is as strategy before structure.

The first decision point is whether to have an ethics committee. Assuming this question is resolved in the affirmative, "ethics" needs to be defined. One may define ethics as a branch of philosophy that deals with the good/bad or right/wrong of behavior as determined by rationality or reason.

The scope of ethics to be dealt with by the committee then needs to be decided. Will it be a clinical or medical ethics committee, dealing only with treatment and other patient issues? Will it address a broad range of issues, including busi ness ethics? Will the committee address internal facility management issues, such as ethical policies and practices? Or will the committee have a broader focus, and include external ethical issues such as those involved in mergers, joint ventures, and new services? It will be helpful both to committee members and to the organization to clarify the scope of ethical issues to be dealt with by the committee.

STATEMENT OF PURPOSE

The purposes of the ethics committee provide it with its charter. The functions of the committee may vary among institutions, and may include any or all of the following:

1) Resource for referral of ethical questions;
2) Policy formulation for recommendations to the governing board of the institution;

3) Education of the staff, patients, families, and the community regarding legal rights and responsibilities; and
4) Case consultation on an individual basis.

POLICY FORMATION

The ethics committee may be called upon to debate policy issues and present recommendations to administration and/or the governing board of the institution. This allows for interdisciplinary dialogue on issues; a process to review and initiate policies; and the opportunity for clinical staff to be involved in policy development. Staff members have found the opportunity to influence those policies which they will have to implement to be a boost to their self-worth.

For example, the Patient Self-Determination Act (PSDA) required a written policy regarding advance directives for each health care institution by December 1, 1991. Ethics committees provided a sounding board to listen to contrasting opinions on such issues as feeding and hydration as "comfort measures." Recommendations were made concerning policy formation, materials to be presented to patients on admission, who should present the issue to the patient and family (i.e., social worker, physician, and/or nursing personnel); forms were drawn for recording the patient's wishes; and suggestions for patient follow-up were made. Discussion regarding many of these issues continues in most facilities.

In establishing the committee, the manner of presentation of the group's consensus should be addressed. Should the ethics committee have the authority to endorse or disagree with facility policy? For example, some facilities have asked the ethics committee to endorse the facility policy regarding advance directives. Included in the intake information given to new admissions may be a statement from the ethics committee "encouraging" individuals to exercise their right of self-determination by executing advance directives.

EDUCATION

The ethics committee may serve as a forum to educate and improve communication for patients, family members, staff, physicians, and the community. Discussion may center around professional or popular literature, current legislative actions, and ethical issues in the news.

A handbook may be developed which describes the ethics committee's role while providing information about common ethical dilemmas in long-term care. The committee may choose to create a library of press clippings, ethics newsletters, legal literature, journal articles, and books. These materials can be made available to residents, family, and staff (Welch,1992).

CASE CONSULTATION

The challenge for the committee members is to manage crisis with proactive solutions. There are several operational questions for an ethics committee doing individual case consultation.

Who should have the right or authority to bring a case to the Ethics Committee? Options may include patients; family members; the legal guardian or agent under a durable power of attorney for health care; attending physician; medical director; facility staff—the director of nursing may serve to screen cases and attempt to resolve situations before they are brought to the committee; or outside interests, e.g., hospices or other agencies. Situations may arise where clergy disagree with the family. There needs to be an acknowledgment of the family's right to be present at the discussion of certain issues.

Are there situations where bringing a case to the ethics

committee should be mandatory? If yes, under what circumstances? Can a case consultation be vetoed before it is heard by the committee and, if so, by whom?

Should the ethics committee take recorded votes in individual cases? Should the group operate by majority vote, by consensus, or by discussion without any attempt to reach a majority vote in consensus? If the group reaches consensus in individual cases, should the decision be binding or advisory on the participants?

Who should be present to hear cases? Should all members participate or only a subcommittee (of what size)? At times, cases may need to be heard quickly. What constitutes a "majority" of members to hear a case? Should a consultant list of persons outside the committee be appointed for specific cases?

There are also questions of confidentiality. *What written records, if any, should the committee create* regarding its consultation in a particular case? *Where should these records be maintained*, and who should have access to them? *What should be placed on the resident's chart? Should the resident's medical record indicate that the ethics committee has been involved in his case*?

Concern arises that the committee might be used to "second-guess" the attending physician. It may be best to let tension and frustration among staff play out in an internal organization, rather then elsewhere. Generally, if staff feel they have a forum, they tend to be more satisfied.

OPERATIONAL ISSUES OF THE COMMITTEE

Committee Membership

The next decision point is the size of the committee. The number of members may vary from 8 to 30. Actually, 10 to 12 provides for a very workable committee. Deciding on the areas of expertise that are wanted on the committee helps to determine the number. Types of persons frequently found on the committee include: Director of Nursing, Medical Director, administrator, social worker, ethicist, pastoral care clergy, attorney, Mission Services, the Board of Trustees, and representatives of other long-term care facilities.

The persons serving on the committee then need to be specified. Deciding the length of terms and a rotation schedule, so that a few new members may be added each year, proves helpful when such planning is done before the committee is established. Also, are members appointed, and by whom? Are members paid, or volunteers? Can members be reappointed and, if so, for how many terms? Our experience is that 2-year terms appointed by the CEO with possible reappointment is effective. Most members of ethics committees are not paid.

It is very helpful in recruiting members of ethics committees to be able to tell them at the outset the frequency and length of meetings. The frequency varies widely; in some organizations, meetings are held monthly, while some hold them quarterly and others hold them every other month. Our experience is that regular meetings held every other month for 1 1/2 hours are effective. Special meetings may be called when there is an immediate issue.

Record Keeping

Minutes of meetings are needed. A secretary for each term can be appointed or members can serve as secretary on a rotating basis. Confidentiality of minutes influences their circulation. One way of maintaining this confidentiality is to have the ethics committee instituted as a subcommittee of the Quality Assurance Committee. Minutes of the meetings are circulated only to the members of the committee. Residents are referenced in the minutes by using their identification numbers instead of names.

Another decision point concerns the committee's reporting relationship. Will it be a Board Committee, an Administrative Committee, or simply an Education Committee? Our experience has been to favor an Administrative Committee making recommendations to the CEO. Quarterly reports are made to the Board of Trustees. Other options include a decisionmaking committee with implementation authority, versus a committee having only an education function.

A decision regarding how the ethics committee fits into the organization provides a functional framework for it. One organizational structure is as follows:

Board of Trustees

CEO/Administrator

Quality Assurance Diretcor

Quality Assurance Committee

Medical Care Subcommittee	Ethics Subcommittee	Utilization Review Subcommittee

Each ethics subcommittee protocol should be reviewed and/or revised every 2 years to ensure its effectiveness.

MODELS OF ETHICS COMMITTEE FUNCTIONING

The following section presents four models for committee functioning.

Pure Committee Model

Members of the committee function as a whole in fulfilling the purpose of the committee. Some feel this is a good starting point, but that the whole group is too large (depending on the number of persons serving on the committee) and is intimidating. Others have found this model very effective, especially if the committee is small.

Subcommittee as Consultant

A subcommittee serves as a consultant on a rotating basis per quarter. Alternatively, a subcommittee can be formed to deal with a specific issue, utilizing the pertinent expertise of the committee members. A committee member can serve as a consultant and is on call to deal with ethical issues as they arise.

Post Facto Committee Review

Ethical issues are brought to the committee after they have been resolved primarily for educational purposes. Both the subcommittee model and the committee model may provide post facto review of cases for the committee as a whole.

Pure Consultation Model

An ethicist is a member of the committee, and this person resolves issues. The goal is to enhance the skills of the committee so that the ethicist works himself/herself out of a job.

PREPARING THE ETHICS COMMITTEE

Preparation of committee members may occur after their appointment and during initial monthly meetings which are purely educational. Topics such as "Ethics and the Law," "Resident Care at End of Life," "Advance Directives," and the hospice philosophy have proved helpful. Members can be sent to workshops on a variety of ethical topics to enhance their knowledge base. Subscriptions to ethics publications such as the *Hastings Center Report, Ethics and Medics, Issues in Law and Medicine*, and others can be helpful as ongoing reference material. If the facility is part of a health system or a regional consortium, ethics education programs may be sponsored and made available by them.

A good way to begin is with policy development. As policies are discussed, ethical issues will be clarified. Initially, ethical issues are usually referred from committee members, but as the organization becomes more aware of the Ethics Committee and its role, referral of issues comes from physicians, residents, family members and staff.

MAINTAINING A FUNCTIONAL ETHICS COMMITTEE

A number of approaches may be implemented to ensure that the committee remains a viable entity in the organization. Some of those that have been successful include:

- *Provision of ongoing educational materials.* Information packets of current articles, workshop materials, and other items can be provided at each meeting.
- *Formation of subcommittees* provides helpful "feed-in" for meetings agendas. Some that have proved useful are: a Policy Subcommittee to draft needed policies; a Resident Review Subcommittee to monitor the Advance Directive status and ethical care issues of residents, and a Forms Subcommittee to develop appropriate forms, e.g., Referral of Ethical Issues Forms and Resident Competency Forms.
- Since many ethical concerns may not reach the committee, a *process to be in touch with current ethical issues in the organization* is helpful. This entails education of staff and physicians regarding the Ethics Committee and its functions, policies regarding the role of the Ethics Committee, and a form for referral of ethical issues.
- A *regular meeting schedule* facilitates the effectiveness of the Ethics Committee. It is helpful if meetings are set for the entire year so committee members can plan to attend; e.g., on the second Friday of every other month, from 12:30—2:00 p.m.
- *An agenda for each meeting* with items prioritized is helpful.
- *Cases to be presented for consultation are written up* to provide the necessary facts in concise form. The ethical question needs to be clearly stated. This facilitates the focus of the committee.
- An ethical decisionmaking process facilitates orderly dis-

cussion and working through of the issues or cases to a rec-
ommendation(s) for action.

COMPARING OBJECTIVES: HOSPITAL VS. NURSING HOME

There are significant differences between the respective
roles of hospital and long-term care facility ethics committees. With an average age of 82 nationwide, the resident
population of nursing homes is much more vulnerable
(Hirsh, 1987).

Time Frame

The time frame during which patients are cared for as
they progress from onset to resolution of an illness is much
longer in a nursing home. Nursing homes generally are not
faced with the need to make decisions about a patient's
medical care with the same speed that is necessary in hospitals (Hirsh, 1987).

The acute care hospital setting is generally responsible
for diagnosis and treatment of illness, with the goal of elim-
inating it in most circumstances and mitigating it in others.
Once maximum benefit has been gained from intensive
therapy, the hospital's involvement ends. Many patients
then need the continued "supportive" care which is provided at the nursing home.

The staff of long-term care facilities is routinely called
upon to care for the chronically ill, as well as the terminally ill. Caring for patients over greater periods of time allows staff to become increasingly involved with the patient
and family, both emotionally and physically. When a patient's status declines, staff who cared for the premorbid
patient must now change their perspective in caring for the
ailing individual. In the case of the terminally ill patient,
the acceptance that "everything possible" has been done to
mitigate illness and that now only "supportive" care is
helpful is equally difficult for the patient, family and staff.

Patient Transfers

Transferring patients between acute and long-term facilities raises many issues. The nursing home staff must weigh the risks versus benefits of transferring a patient from familiar surroundings to an acute care setting. Decisions are made by taking into account the extent of illness, mental status, projection of beneficial outcome, and capabilities of staff to administer treatment at the nursing home (such as IV fluids and breathing treatments), as well as patient and family expectations. Regulations regarding types and extent of treatment, e.g., nutrition and IV fluids, as well as staffing constraints, may play a role in the decisionmaking process. The question of the ambulance ride itself adding further injury or causing decline in the patient's condition must also be addressed.

Interpersonal Relations

Handling individuals on a daily basis may lead to a high degree of empathy. Confidentiality issues may arise as caring staff members become close to their patients.

Physicians play a much more limited role in the care of patients in nursing homes than in hospitals.

Long-term family conflicts may surface. Family members may disagree with the patient or with one another over critical treatment issues. This often places extended care facility staff in an uncomfortable position. For example, the issue of nutrition and hydration as a "comfort measure" frequently raises questions.

Individuals with no surviving family members, or only distant relatives, pose additional potential problems. An individual may live in an extended care facility over a long period of time, during which their mental capabilities may deteriorate from a competent state to an incompetent one. This situation may arise acutely, e.g., through a cerebral vascular accident, or gradually over time. The home is then left with the responsibility of making legal, financial, and ethical decisions for the patient, unless some form of public or volunteer guardian system is available.

A MODEL FOR THE DECISIONMAKING PROCESS

As with the physical sciences, ethics weighs and analyzes relevant factors before reaching publicly defensible conclusions. The following is a model for reaching ethical decisions that an ethics committee may employ (Drane, 1986).

1) *Identify the Decisionmakers.* Ethics involves variable interests, intuitions, and feelings present in every person concerned with the patient. Experienced clinicians have a great advantage in making ethically defensible judgments. Society and public interests may have their own expression of right and wrong. One can identify goods and values initially by sampling the feelings of different participants. Persons' sensitivities are important ethical considerations.

2) *Consider Relevant Facts.* Diagnosis, prognosis, medical alternatives, and treatment or nontreatment consequences are all important considerations in making a good ethical decision. The right or wrong way to proceed may emerge if all parties thoroughly understand the medical situation.

The human facts to consider include patient competence and mental condition (e.g., depression), religious beliefs of the patient and institution, family situation, and economic issues.

3) *Examine Viable Options.* Facts developed must be ordered into analytic categories. The ethical decision involved must be defined within a specific category, e.g., death, suicide, euthanasia, right to treatment, refusal of treatment, or informed consent. Distinctions should be drawn among available options, e.g., prolonging life and prolonging death, or direct and indirect killing. Accepted ethical principles may be applied to guide in decisionmaking, e.g., re-

spect for life, autonomy, beneficence, justice, and truth. Opinions from legal decisions and professional codes or statements previously written may be used for guidance.

4) *Consider Short-Term and Long-Term Consequences.* Decisions must retain public confidence and be defensible. Outcomes should be predicted to the best of one's ability, based on prior experience and judgment.

5) *List the Values Reflected in the Case.* Broad categories may be used to categorize ethical principles. Widely accepted principles may include justice, truth, beneficence, and respect for life.

6) *Determine the Values in Conflict.* Ethical reflection may be guided by expressing those values in conflict as well as those to which all parties are in agreement.

7) *Prioritize the Values in Light of the Alternatives.* Professional persons making ethical decisions should try to recognize their personal underlying beliefs and to admit their influence on decisions. One must correlate the reasons for supporting one decision over another.

8) *Justify the Decision.* Medical persons should be prepared to explain how professional choices are based on publicly accepted standards of behavior. Professional persons defend themselves by providing reasons for their choices.

CASE EXAMPLES

This chapter next presents an exercise to give readers the experience of analyzing and discussing cases following a protocol. Using the following clinical case histories, the task of an ethics committee would be to reach a consensus by following an established protocol. To assist in the decisionmaking process, several questions have been added specific to each case.

CASE

AZ is a 74-year-old white female who was active and in good health until approximately 6 months prior to arrival at the nursing home. She first noted fatigue and anorexia followed by rapid weight loss, going from 134 pounds to 114 pounds over a 2–3 month period. By the time she reported to her physician, she had developed right upper quadrant pain. A CT scan of the abdomen revealed a mass at the head of the pancreas suspicious for carcinoma. The patient was hospitalized for evaluation. At surgery, she was found to have extensive spread of pancreatic carcinoma which was unresectable and untreatable. A tube was placed in the biliary duct to drain secretions externally. The patient and family were informed of the terminal prognosis, with life expectancy predicted less than 6 months. The patient was a widow with two sons living in close proximity. The patient and her family elected for nursing home placement in view of her projected needs for total care. With the advice of their physician, all agreed to proceed on a plan of supportive care only.

On admission to the home, the patient was pleasant, with full mental capacity, ambulatory with assistance, and able to eat fairly well. She remained stable for approximately 2 months. During that time, the staff came to know and like her. She was talkative, always smiling, and seldom complained.

Her decline over the next 2 months was painfully slow and unremitting. She had constant pain, progressive anorexia, and marked pruritus (itching from a buildup of toxins). Somehow, the patient managed to maintain her pleasant disposition, and rarely complained. At this point, the tube which had been draining biliary secretions dislodged and fell out.

What should be done to comfort this dying patient? In order to replace the tube, the patient would need transport back to the hospital where the procedure could be done as an outpatient under CT guidance. The trip would be painful, and there was no guarantee of success. If not replaced, her secretions would continue to accumulate, causing increased confusion and eventual coma (hepatic encephalopathy). The patient was no longer mentally able to participate in the decision. After multiple discussions between the family and their physician, the decision was made not to attempt replacement. One son was in full agreement, while the other was unsure about the decision.

Several days passed as the patient was observed by staff to have intense pain partially relieved by increasing doses of morphine and increasing periods of agitation. Her oral intake was minimal. The director of nursing was approached by several staff members and urged to take action to help the patient.

SPECIFIC QUESTIONS TO ADDRESS IN THE DECISIONMAKING PROCESS

1. Does the facility have a policy regarding this element of care/treatment? What are the legal ramifications of not following the policy of the facility?

2. What factors influenced the patient and/or family's decision, e.g., beliefs, values, mental impairment, physical impairment, depression, pain, or wish to die?

3. Does the family understand what it means to refuse treatment?

4. What is the effect of the different alternatives on staff morale?

CASE

GT is a 91-year-old white male who was in excellent health until approximately 10 months prior to admission. He had suffered no major illness during his lifetime and continued to play golf until he began developing shortness of breath. A full evaluation including bronchoscopy revealed pulmonary fibrosis. Treatment options were limited. The patient was quite frustrated with his lack of endurance and change in lifestyle.

Approximately 6 months later, the patient noted some rectal bleeding. A barium enema revealed a probable rectal carcinoma. The patient was reluctant to proceed with surgery, since he was told a colostomy would be required.

Two months later, he suffered a severe cerebral vascular accident. He was left with complete left-sided hemiparesis, aphasia (inability to talk), and dysphagia (dysfunctional swallowing). The patient was alert and able to eat small quantities. Following intensive rehabilitation efforts in the hospital, the patient was discharged to the nursing home for continued therapy. He had no further return of motor function and showed signs of depression.

Shortly after his admission to the nursing home, he began to develop symptoms of bowel obstruction. Eating was painful with frequent emesis and aspiration. The patient and family refused surgical considerations and did not want feeding tubes or IV hydration. After approximately 1 week, the patient developed pneumonia presumed secondary to aspiration.

The case was brought to the ethics committee by the patient's son, who requested no treatment and comfort measures only.

SPECIFIC QUESTIONS TO ADDRESS IN THE DECISIONMAKING PROCESS

1) Does the facility have a policy regarding this element of care/treatment? What are the legal ramifications of not following the policy of the facility?

2) What factors influenced the resident and/or family's decision, e.g., beliefs, values, mental impairment, physical impairment, depression, pain, or wish to die?

3) Does the patient and/or family understand what it means to refuse treatment?

4) What is the effect of the different alternatives on staff morale?

SUMMARY

The information presented here should serve as a stimulus to those faced with the task of developing and continually refining their ethics committees. An Ethics Committee provides a promising inhouse structure to negotiate the ethical pressures exerted by new technology. An interdisciplinary, rational dialogue can be established to deal with ethical issues and support the administration, family members, physicians, and staff who struggle with them.

Advantages of Ethics Committees in Long-Term Care

An Ethics Committee makes a real contribution to the life of the facility. It does so by:

- Providing an ethical resource in the facility;
- Promoting ethics education in the facility and the community;
- Facilitating ethical inquiry and legitimizing the raising of ethical issues;
- Supporting those with ethical concerns;
- Resolving conflicts; and
- Resolving issues prior to legal involvement.

Dangers or Risks of Ethics Committees

The advantages of ethics committees far outweigh the risks. Some of the potential disadvantages may include:

- Interference with the doctor/patient relationship;
- Taking over decisionmaking inappropriately;
- Group-think (a dominant person decides); or
- Protection of the institution rather than openly dealing with issues.

While any of these scenarios may conceivably occur, a well-thought-through protocol for the Ethics Committee makes any or all of these potential dangers extremely unlikely.

REFERENCES

Drane, J. F. (1986). A methodology for making ethical health care decisions. *Health Progress, 10*, 36–37, 64.

Drane, J. F., & Roth, R. B. (1985). Institutional ethics committees: What, how, and why. *Health Progress, 10*, 30–34, 56.

Hirsh, H. L. (1987). Nursing home ethics committees: To be or not to be. *Nursing Homes, 5/6*, 12–15.

Welch, R. M. (1992). Ethics committees provide decisionmaking support. *Provider, 11*, 49.

The Patient Self-Determination Act in the Home Care Setting

4

Amy Marie Haddad, Ph.D., R.N., C.

The federal Patient Self-Determination Act (PSDA) passed as part of the Omnibus Budget Reconciliation Act (OBRA) of 1990 and became effective December 1, 1991. It applies to all health care institutions, including home care programs, that participate in Medicare and Medicaid. As home care providers work to comply with the requirements of the PSDA, they confront the substantial differences that exist between home care and traditional institutional settings, such as hospitals and nursing homes, in relation to health care decisionmaking. The purpose of this chapter is to examine what the implementation of the PSDA means in the context of home care. The chapter also explores selected ethical and practical implications of the PSDA in this context. Finally, areas for research and reflective inquiry are proposed.

OVERVIEW OF PSDA REQUIREMENTS

The United States Congress passed the Patient Self-Determination Act in response to a variety of social, legal, and political influencing factors. The act requires hospitals, home health care agencies, skilled nursing facilities, and hospice programs receiving Medicare and Medicaid funds to inform patients of their rights under state law to execute advance directives such as living wills, durable powers of attorney for health care decisions, and other forms of proxy decisionmaking.

Four specific actions are mandated by the PSDA:

1) assessing on admission and documenting in the patient's medical record concerning whether or not an advance directive exists;

2) offering adult patients written information and summaries of institutional policies concerning their ability under state law to accept or reject treatment;

3) informing patients of their right to execute an advance directive; and

4) providing educational programs about advance directives to the institution's staff and the community (Omnibus Budget Reconciliation Act [OBRA] 1990).

These initial requirements provided little in the way of specific instructions. Health care providers did not receive further clarification of the law until March, 1992, when the Health Care Financing Administration (HCFA) published its interim final rule (57 *Federal Register* 8194–8204 [6 March 1992]). However, the interim final rule does little to clarify the original act's intent. It seems merely to reinforce the requirements to inform patients of state law regarding directives, document existing directives in the medical record, and educate the community. HCFA has left it to providers to fully develop and implement these requirements.

The underlying goals of the PSDA are ambitious, ambiguous, and questionably attainable. One goal of the statute is to encourage, but not require, adults to complete advance directives: "Advance directives have been proposed to answer the problem of how to empower patients so that they maintain control of their care even when incompetent"

(Lynn & Teno, 1993, p. 23). Another unspoken goal is to prompt health care providers to honor advance directives. This goal seems to be closest to the intention of the original sponsors of the act, Senators John C. Danforth (R-Mo.) and Daniel Patrick Moynihan (D-N.Y.), who wanted to empower people to take part in the decisions that affect their lives and to correct the balance of the relationship between health care consumers and providers (McCloskey, 1991).

A third goal is to avoid the use of the courts as an arbiter in decisions regarding termination of life-sustaining treatment in the case of incompetent patients. The idea behind this goal is to prevent tragic struggles between family members, health care professionals, lawyers, and administrators concerning the withdrawing or withholding of life-sustaining treatment in the case of an incompetent patient. Furthermore, formal advance directives provide the "clear and convincing evidence" required in some states to discontinue life-sustaining treatment. The successful implementation of all of these goals remains to be seen.

Home care providers, as well as providers in other settings, are left with the task of interpreting the letter and intent of the law. Home care providers approach this task with no small amount of apprehension due to past experience with the vagaries of federal regulations. HCFA has not been specific about *who* must receive information about advance directives; *when* this information must be given; *how* and *when* to document this information; and *how* home care providers are supposed to comply when advance directives conflict with agency policy. However, home care providers suspect that they will be held accountable for these details (Sabatino, 1993). The statute does not distinguish among the various practice settings to which a patient might be admitted. It is as if the admission processes to a hospice program, hospital, nursing home, or home care program were uniform. Clearly, each setting requires a different spin on the implementation of the PSDA, and the context of home care is no exception.

CONTEXT OF HOME CARE

Before one can begin a discussion of the implementation of the PSDA in the home care context, it is important to clarify what home care is. During the last decade, home care has been the fastest growing sector of the health care system. Treating people at home is generally cost-effective, provides a psychological lift and greater opportunity for activity and participation in family life, and enhances the wellbeing and autonomy of patients. Home care may sound simple and domestic, but the changes in services, type of client, products, and reimbursement complicate and confound home care practice.

Although state licensure laws specifically delineate the requirements of a "home care agency," the home care marketplace is swamped with providers of numerous services and products, all of which could be called "home care." Thus, it seems that the definition of home care can change depending on whom one asks. The following discussion provides an overview of the most common types of formal services and products provided under the rubric of home care:

- *Home Medical Equipment.* Comprises everything from ambulatory aids to wheelchairs to incontinence supplies to respiratory equipment such as ventilators and oxygen. Home medical equipment includes disposable items such as dressings and durable items, such as a hospital bed, that are generally rented on a per diem basis.
- *Home Parenteral/Enteral Services.* Includes intravenous therapies such as chemotherapy, antibiotics, blood products, and total parenteral nutrition, as well as enteral solutions and pumps for gastrostomy feeding.
- *Public Health Nursing.* Provides traditional community health services, such as instruction about nutrition and hygiene. Public health nursing is largely involved with preventive care and maternal/child health, such as prenatal and postnatal visits.
- *Medicare.* Comprises a large percentage of home care services. It is defined as care in the home that is intermittent and skilled (nursing and rehabilitation services) for home-

bound patients who are eligible for Medicare benefits (generally those 65 and over).

- *Home Uterine Monitoring.* Manages premature contractions with medications and monitors in the home.
- Hospice. A care philosophy for terminal patients that can be provided in the home or an institutional setting.
- *Home Phototherapy.* Provides treatment for hyperbilirubinemia for premature infants.
- *Private Duty Nursing.* Provides skilled nursing services outside the purview of Medicare. Private duty nursing can be provided on a round-the-clock basis for highly complex patients in lieu of hospitalization.
- Home Health Aide/Homemaker Services. Provides services and care that are considered "unskilled" in that they do not require licensure but are commonly provided in concert with skilled services. Services that a home health aide might provide include light meal preparation and basic physical care, such as bathing and grooming. Homemaker services include light housekeeping and chore service such as minor repairs to the home.
- Home Rehabilitation. Includes the services provided by physical, occupational, and speech therapists, and vocational therapy.

Regardless of the variety of services and products provided in home care, the core aspects of home care can be distilled to the following four categories: 1) nursing care which includes assessment, interventions and teaching; 2) home medical equipment and supplies; 3) drugs; and 4) rehabilitation services. It is probable that the competitive home care provider of the future will offer all four components. Presently, home care services and products are offered to patients in piecemeal fashion, often requiring the coordination of three or four separate home care providers in the care of a single patient.

Differences Between Home Care and Institutional Care

First, the question of who is responsible for obtaining information from the patient regarding advance directives in an institution has been difficult enough to resolve. The multiplicity of home care providers involved in a single case complicates the question of responsibility further. For example, in a hospital the responsibility might fall with the patient representative, the physician, or the nurse. In the case of a hospital, all of the members of the health care team work within the same facility and share a single patient medical record.

In home care, the assignment of responsibility for informing the patient about advance directives is made more difficult when one considers the number of home care agencies and their respective employees involved in a patient's care. Not only do home care providers have to decide who is responsible *within* their agency for informing patients about advance directives and documenting their existence, but they must also coordinate responsibility between cooperating agencies.

The PSDA guarantees that all patients admitted to home care will get information about advance directives. However, it is unlikely that the statute intends that patients be asked about advance directives repeatedly by all of the different home care providers that enter a patient's home. On the other hand, home care providers must guard against the assumption that someone else has asked the patient about advance directives when, in fact, no one has.

Second, the regulatory issues governing home care providers, though increasingly cumbersome, are quite different from those applicable to nursing homes and hospitals and have a significant impact on decisionmaking. Regardless of the degree of regulation governing home care practice, home care remains essentially hidden from public and professional eyes. The actions of a home care provider regarding advance directives are more private than those in an institution. The isolation of home care has been cause for concern about the vulnerability of frail patients. Thus, home care providers may need to be more cautious about protecting a patient's right and documenting discussions about health care decision making.

Third, the informed consent doctrine does not precisely fit into the home setting. Generally, home care is less focused than acute care on specific, cure-oriented treatment. Home care is basically chronic care, so decisionmaking is more concerned with plans for care throughout the course of an illness, rather than the avoidance of loss of control while dying and incompetent. The very setting of home care may make patients less fearful about losing control over treatment decisions, since care delivery takes place on the patient's "turf." At home, patients may feel more secure and willing to assert their rights. Attempts to override patient wishes in the home are likely to be perceived as a direct attack on independence.

Finally, home care differs most markedly and simply from institutional care in the site where care is delivered. Home care is delivered in a patient's home. A home is generally not equipped with the latest life-sustaining technology. However, high-tech, "user-friendly," and safe equipment has permitted the introduction of a variety of treatment and mechanical supports in the home. High-tech home care includes the use of volume ventilators, parenteral and enteral access devices, and dialysis. What is different about the use of these sophisticated types of equipment in the home, as opposed to the hospital or nursing home, is that their use must be negotiated with the patient and his or her family. The technological imperative, i.e., the demand to use equipment merely because it is easily available, is not as strong in home care for the practical reason that a conscious decision must be made to bring health care technology into the home.

Thus, even before the passage of the PSDA, home care providers traditionally discussed contingencies for care with the patient and the family *before* admission. This was done to realistically plan for service delivery and to decide what equipment and treatment were appropriate to match mutually agreed upon goals. The most significant differences between an institutional care setting and home care may be stated as follows (Collopy, Dubler & Zuckerman, 1990):

> Homes are not hospitals. They are not designed as settings for caregiving. They become such only reactively, incrementally, and often under duress, as illness and frailty invade the precincts of daily life. Even then, the regimens of care contend with a setting shaped by the personal tastes, fiscal means, and life style of the care recipient. Setting is, then, both a strength and a source of tension in home care. (p. S3)

The tension between the care provider and the care recipient, the duty to do good and the patient's right to autonomy, is discussed further in the section below on ethical implications of the PSDA.

THE HOME CARE ADMISSION PROCESS BEFORE THE PSDA

To highlight the difference the PSDA has made in the admission process in home care, a complex case is presented and discussed in terms of the home care provider's responsibilities before and after the passage of the statute.

CASE

Ms. P, a 62–year-old woman with metastatic breast cancer, had exhausted standard treatment for her disease. However, she wanted to pursue some form of therapy, so she accepted a standard-dose, five-day regimen of leucovorin and 5–fluorouracil. Ms. P discussed her wishes regarding resuscitation and life-sustaining treatment with her primary physician while she was in the hospital. The physician wrote a "do-not-resuscitate" (DNR) order on Ms. P's medical record. Ms. P completed therapy and was scheduled to be discharged to home care. Ms. P didn't have a written advance directive. She had one sister who lived in the same community. Ms. P's sister was disabled but interested in her sister's welfare even if she was unable to assist with her care.

In the days before the passage of the PSDA, the home care provider would have planned for Ms. P's discharge to home care by completing a comprehensive patient assessment. This assessment would include information about Ms. P's goals for and expectations from home care. The home care provider would have discussed a number of contingencies with Ms. P to discern just what she wanted regarding treatment should her status change. For example, it would have been every bit as important to discuss a "do-not-hospitalize" decision with Ms. P as it would a "do-not-resuscitate" decision. To the extent it is possible to predict while competent what one would want when and if one were to become incompetent, the prudent home care provider would have assisted Ms. P to make such a prediction.

The home care provider would have emphasized that Ms. P was free to change her mind at any time. A consent form or contract outlining the general terms of home care service delivery was commonly used to initiate home care.

The home care provider, in conjunction with Ms. P's attending physician, would then have developed a detailed plan of care for all of the members of the health care team involved in Ms. P's care including her wishes to forego further treatment; i.e., whether or not to initiate cardiopulmonary resuscitation in the event of a cardiac or pulmonary arrest, whether or not to call the emergency medical system, and whether or not to hospitalize and for what reasons. For example, Ms. P might not have wanted to be hospitalized for more chemotherapy, but probably would have wanted to be hospitalized for insertion of an intravenous access device for easier administration of pain medication.

These types of informal advance directives were very common in home care and were adapted to the needs of the patient and family. This initial care plan often reflected the first of many discussions regarding decisions about care and changed as a patient's illness progressed.

HOME CARE ADMISSION PROCESS AFTER
THE PSDA

In the post-PSDA era, given the same history, diagnosis, and prognosis as part of the comprehensive admission assessment, the home care provider is required by law to specifically inquire about advance directives for Ms. P as with all adult patients admitted to home care. Since Ms. P had a DNR order, the home care provider would know that some discussion about advance directives has occurred. Let us assume Ms. P does not have a formal advance directive. The home care provider is then required to inform the patient about his or her right to complete a formal advance directive. Furthermore, the home care provider is obligated to share written information regarding the home care agency's policies and procedures concerning Ms. P's ability under state law to accept or reject treatment. This information should include an overview of agency policies on foregoing life-sustaining treatment. Ms. P should be made to understand that an advance directive is a way to express her preferences, whatever they may be.

The home care agency should have a formal policy for documenting the presence or absence of an advance directive in the patient's permanent medical record. These advance directives should also be a part of the plan of care and shared with all relevant staff who will be caring for Ms. P in the home, to ensure that her wishes are carried out. Since Ms. P does have a living relative in the community, the home care provider might wish to contact her as well, with Ms. P's permission. It would be up to Ms. P to decide if she would like to involve her sister more, such as by making her sister a formal proxy decisionmaker. In any case, for practical and humane reasons it is important to inform the family, with the patient's permission, about treatment decisions.

If Ms. P had previously executed an advance directive, the home care provider should do more than note its existence. The home care provider should obtain, review and discuss it with the patient and recommend a clearer or more specific document if need be. If the advance directive is a durable power of attorney for health care decisions, the home care provider should inquire if the proxy decisionmaker named in the document has been notified of the patient's wishes regarding treatment or nontreatment. Pinch and Parsons (1992) noted in a study of healthy non-institutionalized elderly (N=20):

> Although a number of individuals had developed living wills and appointed proxies, many had failed to notify the individual that they had been placed in such a role. If notified, some had not necessarily discussed their desires about treatments with the potential proxy. (p. 21)

In order to fulfill his or her obligations as a proxy, i.e., to represent the wishes of the incompetent patient and work with the home care team as the situation unfolds, the proxy must be informed.

It is evident from the preceding examples that the introduction of the PSDA requires more formalized, extensive discussions with patients and their proxies, as well as clearer documentation.

Additionally, home care providers are required to provide education and training to their personnel and the community. Some providers have chosen to comply with this portion of the statute by holding inservice educational sessions that review state law and agency policies. In addition to general education sessions for all employees, some home care providers have focused on the training of an elite few among their personnel—such as the clinical supervisor or admission coordinator, who is frequently a registered nurse or social worker—to deal with all admissions in the area of advance directives. It is unclear what the statute requires in the way of community education. Certainly, by asking every adult admission about advance directives a degree of community education is occurring by default.

IMPLEMENTATION OF THE PSDA IN HOME CARE

In the context of home care, the content, form, and process of decisionmaking about care in general and life-sustaining treatments in particular is complex and varied. The PSDA has qualitatively changed the way home care providers work with patients in making these important choices. The following sections examine the ethical underpinnings of the PSDA and specific challenges unique to the home care setting.

Ethical Implications

Although the PSDA is a legal statute, it is more fully understood in light of the ethical principles that are the foundation of the law. All of the requirements of the PSDA reflect the hallmark of ethically sound decisionmaking in that the PSDA enables competent and informed patients to reach voluntary decisions about their care. The PSDA sets the stage for the patient's quest for self-determination regarding such matters as informed consent for treatment, designation of a surrogate decisionmaker, or the right to accept or refuse life-sustaining treatment. The right to self-determination has its ethical justification in the principle of respect for autonomy.

Respect for autonomy is derived from the broader principle of respect for persons that asserts human beings are unconditionally worthy agents. If human beings are worthy of respect, then it follows that they should be free to choose how they would like to live their lives and make their own decisions without undue interference. Autonomy is central to the intent of the PSDA and reflects the high value placed on it in American society. "Knowing that we are 'the captains of our fate', rather than surmising that we are the pawns of another (no matter how benevolent that other might be), is what most adults, at least in Western culture, want" (Loewy, 1991, p. 156).

Respect for autonomy in an institutional setting is often eroded. The life of an institution is driven by routines. Institutions and their policies often decide what the patient may eat, whom she may see, when he rises, and when he sleeps. Making competent patients part of the decisionmaking process and giving them the final say is accepted in home care not only because it is proper procedure, but also because of the setting of care delivery. Home care is often chosen as a treatment setting so that the patient can regain his or her lost autonomy or prevent the loss of autonomy by delaying the admission to a nursing home. Thus, home care patients enter the patient/provider relationship on more equal footing than they do in an institution. Seen in this light, the PSDA is just one more component of the numerous negotiations necessary to provide care in the home.

Even though the home is not an institution, the introduction of formal home care services sets the stage for potential conflicts between a patient's individual autonomy and the home care provider's legal and ethical responsibilities to provide care. Young, Pignatello, & Taylor (1988) in an empirical study of ethical problems in home care noted that patients often strongly assert their autonomy and are more likely to resist orders or take advice in the home setting than an institution. Home care providers, even though visitors in the patient's home, are in a position to enhance or inhibit patient autonomy while at the same time fulfilling professional obligations.

Respect for autonomy requires that we accept that competent, informed patients have the right to choose from a variety of options and can also decline all treatment. The key element here is that patients require information about treatment options in order to choose intelligently. The home care provider should not assume because a patient is admitted from the hospital or nursing home to home care he or she is well-informed regarding directives.

Discussions about advance directives should not be limited to living wills and durable powers of attorney for health care documents. The home care provider should teach patient and family about what treatment means in clear, understandable terms. The PSDA requires that the home care provider distribute written information regarding 1) a summary of individual rights under State law to make decisions regarding medical care and 2) the policies of the home care provider regarding implementation of those rights. If the home care agency does not have such a policy in place, it will have to draft one. This may be more difficult for home care providers than for large institutions, since home care agencies rarely have the expertise, such as that found in an institutional ethics committee, to address these concerns fully. This written information should be developed at a simple reading level. Studies of informed consent forms show that these forms do not necessarily give patients a clear understanding of the proposed procedure. For example, a review of the readability of consent forms used in pediatric medical research found that they typically require reading skills at the advanced college level (Tarnowski, Allen, Mayhall, & Kelly, 1990).

Home care providers may be concerned about the amount of time that will be required to counsel each patient. An initial discussion of advance directives can be facilitated by a structured set of questions regarding various treatment/non-treatment options, e.g., DNR, administration of artificial food and fluids, and pain management. Some will find that these initial discussions take longer than anticipated due to patient questions and confusion about the efficacy of certain treatments. Further discussion is almost always necessary in any case as the patient's status changes.

The discussion about advance directives may or may not prompt a patient to execute one. It is possible that a sizable number of patients may wish to complete an advance directive. In a study of 74 homebound patients who were counseled about durable power of attorney, 48 completed one (Markson & Steel, 1990). However, in a randomized controlled trial of an educational intervention regarding advance directives, Sachs and colleagues found that 85% of the patients in the study did not execute a living will (Sachs, Stocking, & Miles, 1992). The PSDA does not instruct a home care provider in handling instances in which the patient wishes to execute an advance directive. A home care agency is neither required to assist, nor is it prohibited from providing assistance to patients wishing to prepare such a document. The home care agency will have to decide for itself to what degree it advocates for the completion of advance directives, based on the agency's philosophy and available resources.

Patients can also "choose not to choose," i.e., choose not to be involved in the decisionmaking process. Choosing not to choose is as legitimate a choice as any other and should be honored (Loewy, 1989). In this type of case, the patient might, for example, choose to do whatever the "doctor recommends." The patient should be notified that physicians generally cannot be legal proxies for their patients. If the patient is reluctant to participate in decisionmaking, the home care provider should recommend that the patient appoint a formal proxy decisionmaker.

Additional ethical principles helpful in analyzing the PSDA are beneficence and nonmaleficence. The principle of beneficence holds that we have a positive duty, dependent on relationship, to do good. The corollary principle of nonmaleficence requires that we avoid harm. Nonmaleficence is not dependent on relationship, i.e., we owe this duty not to do harm to others at all times. Beneficence as an ethical principle is integral to the PSDA. Before the home care provider can do good for the patient, the "good" must be determined. The biomedical good, in pursuit of which patients seek out medical care (for the purposes of the present discussion, home care), is seen as only one (and not necessarily the highest) in a hierarchy of personal goods (Pellegrino & Thomasma, 1988).

The PSDA assumes that advance directives are a "good" and therefore should be encouraged. Although home care providers may not agree with the usefulness of advance directives, by law they must inquire whether or not the patient has one. It is important for the home care provider to know what patients think they are doing and what they have accomplished in making or completing an advance directive.

As the home care provider works with the patient to understand advance directives, specific preferences should be explored, especially where they are apparently not sensible and consistent with previously stated values. In so doing, it is important to avoid forcing one's own vision of the "good" upon a patient.

Since home care providers are required to ask every new patient, they may find cultures or cohorts who find the idea of advance directives repugnant or ludicrous. For example, some question if it is really necessary to ask adults with curable, limited disorders about treatment decisions in the remote event they become incompetent. The PSDA does not distinguish between terminal and essentially healthy adult patients, so all must be routinely asked. It is possible that some harm, or at a minimum some emotional distress, could come to relatively healthy patients who are asked about advance directives. This argument assumes that advance planning is only relevant to the very sick and old. However, "Planning with young, healthy patients may be considered analogous to screening for illness; the chance of illness is low, but the effort may be worth it" (Emanuel, 1991, p. S6). Thus, in the long run these discussions may do good by educating the public about this option for future decisionmaking.

Finally, the principle of fidelity also influences the implementation of advance directives. Fidelity, or faithfulness, includes obligations to be truthful and to keep promises (Ross, 1930). Home care providers must make sure that they fully understand patient wishes before promising they will be carried out. The home care provider must guard against the belief that the work is done when the advance directive is formally written and safely in the chart. The work really comes in faithfully executing the advance directives. Often home care providers are the only outside contacts a patient has. The duty of fidelity weighs particularly heavy in these cases.

SPECIFIC CHALLENGES IN HOME CARE

The implementation of the PSDA in home care has been met with barriers and conflicts. Although the following challenges are not unique to home care, the context of care requires a different perspective and response.

Terminally Ill Patients

Home care providers are often confronted with patients who are terminally ill and have chosen their homes as the setting for their deaths. The home care provider must work closely with the patient's physician in these cases to clarify advance directives. Physicians with little experience in home care may not understand the limits of the setting and have unrealistic expectations of care in the home.

It is up to the home care provider to clarify the wishes of the patient so that the physician understands and can order appropriate care. Ideally, the physician's orders should emanate from full discussion between patient, home care provider, and physician. "It should be emphasized that only a licensed physician—and not the home care agency acting independently—may enter a valid 'do not' order" (Haddad & Kapp, 1991, p. 94).

Patients who are terminally ill, have explored and exhausted active treatment options, and have decided to die at home, should have some idea about life support systems and treatment, so that they may be better able to decide. However, many terminally ill patients will not be well-prepared to make good medical decisions. The same care and attention should be paid to the terminally ill in planning for care in the event of their possible incompetence as to other patients.

Incompetent Patients

Home care providers are required to ask all adult patients about advance directives. The PSDA makes no provision for distributing written information to an adult patient who is admitted or initially comes under care while mentally incompetent. One of the general criteria for admission to home care is the ability to function safely in the home environment with the assistance of formal services. It would be unlikely that an incompetent patient would be admitted to home care without some type of substitute decisionmaker. The home care provider would then work with this substitute decisionmaker in planning care.

The more likely scenario is that a patient will *become* incompetent after admission to home care. It is for just such an eventuality that advance directives are drawn.

Previous competently made directives may work against present incompetent interests (Robertson, 1991). The home care provider, in concert with the patient and his or her physician, should discuss what factors should be considered in making decisions. The home care provider needs to know how strictly an individual patient wants advance directives followed. For example, 150 mentally competent dialysis patients were interviewed regarding their life-sustaining treatment choices. While 88% of the subjects agreed that they wanted pain and suffering to be considered by their proxy decisionmakers, they also wanted their quality of life considered (Sehgal, Galbraith, Chesney, Schoenfeld, Charles, & Lo, 1992). Advance directives should be periodically re-evaluated in light of these qualifications.

Conflicts with the Family

Families play pivotal roles in home care and are often involved in direct caregiving. Even if family members are unable to participate directly, they offer help with "nonmedical" needs such as house maintenance and business affairs. Personal autonomy of the patient in home care can be helped or hindered by family members. Family members may give directives to home care providers that run counter to those of the patient.

Regardless of the presence or absence of an advance directive, the following scenario is not uncommon in home care: The patient becomes incompetent as she or he nears an anticipated death in the home. The patient has a cardiopulmonary arrest. Rather than following through with the patient's wishes to die at home, the family often panics and calls for emergency assistance. Once the emergency medical system is initiated, it is almost impossible to stop the process. Emergency medical technicians are required to make every effort to resuscitate a patient. The patient's advance planning and, worse, his or her wishes are ignored as the patient is rushed to a hospital, often to die in the emergency room. The home care provider will not always be able to prevent this type of occurrence. However, anticipatory teaching with the family members may help prepare them for the death of their loved one and reduce the anxiety that accompanies the event. Families should be counseled repeatedly that treatment directives should not be overridden lightly.

Conflicts With Values

What happens when a member of the home care team, most likely the nurse who is delivering direct care, has ethical or religious conflicts with a patient's advance directive? For example, a nurse may have concerns about withholding nutrition and hydration from a patient in accord with advance directives. These objections should be voiced to the supervisor in the home care agency. The dilemma could be resolved by reassignment or other methods if the nurse and supervisor are willing to compromise. The patient's right to refuse treatment must be balanced against the deeply held convictions of the personnel involved.

Just as many patients haven't given a great deal of thought to advance directives, so, too, home care personnel may not have fully articulated their feelings about withholding and withdrawing treatment until they are confronted with a specific patient who challenges their values. Staff should be given the opportunity to share their feelings and concerns in training about advance directives in addition to procedural information about the PSDA.

EVALUATION

Perhaps the least defined and most challenging aspect of the PSDA is in the area of evaluation. The basic question is whether or not the PSDA is doing any good. Research is needed in a variety of areas to answer this general question and more specific ones regarding the PSDA. The attitudes of home care patients and providers toward advance directives require increased attention. Who should initiate the discussion, where should it take place, and when? What kind of training for staff and patients do we need?

One could diminish the PSDA to another bureaucratic process, merely a check mark on an admission sheet—does discussion of advance directives flow from the mission of the home care provider? Does it make a difference in the number of completed advance directives?

Reevaluation with patients regarding advance directives should be monitored to establish if, and how often, the topic should be revisited in home care. Often the relationship in home care is prolonged and constant. The home care provider is not only forced to deal with issues of a prolonged relationship, but also of a deep one which might obscure objectivity. Should care providers who are not as intimately involved with the patient revisit the question? Are patients treated differently with or without advance directives?

Finally, what effect(s) do advance directives have on home care? In an often cited study by Schneiderman et al. of 204 patients with life-threatening illnesses, the authors found that advance directives had no significant positive or negative effect on a patient's wellbeing, health status, medical treatments, or medical treatment charges (Schneiderman, Kronick, Kaplan, Anderson, & Langer, 1992). This type of study needs to be replicated in the home care environment. Such research would provide substance for educating home care providers, guidance for effective and efficient implementation of the PSDA, and insight into practical ways to improve patient care while concurrently honoring advance directives.

REFERENCES

Collopy, B., Dubler, N., & Zuckerman, C. (1990). The ethics of home care: Autonomy and accommodation. *The Hastings Center Report, 20*(2) S1–S16.

Emanuel, L. (1991). PSDA in the clinic. *Hastings Center Report, 21*(5), S6–S7.

Haddad, A. M., & Kapp, M. B. (1991). *Ethical and legal issues in home health care.* Norwalk, CT: Appleton and Lange.

Loewy, E. H. (1989). *Textbook of medical ethics.* New York: Plenum Publishers.

Loewy, E. H. (1991). Involving patients in Do Not Resuscitate (DNR) decisions: An old issue raising its ugly head. *Journal of Medical Ethics, 17* 156–160.

Lynn, J., & Teno, J. M. (1993). After the Patient Self-Determination Act: The need for empirical research on formal advance directives. *The Hastings Center Report 23*, 20–23.

Markson, L., & Steel, K. (1990). Using advance directives in the home-care setting: A pilot project. *Generations, 14* 25–29.

McCloskey, E. (1991). The Patient Self-Determination Act. *Kennedy Institute of Ethics Journal, 1*, 163–169.

Omnibus Budget Reconcilation Act of 1990. Public Law no. 101–508, H.R. 5834 (November 1990).

Pellegrino, E. D., & Thomasma, D. C. (1988). *For the patient's good: The restoration of beneficence in health care.* New York: Oxford University Press.

Pinch, W. J., & Parsons, M. E. (1992). The patient self-determination act: The ethical dimensions. *Nurse Practioner Forum, 3*, 16–22.

Robertson, J. A. (1991). Second thoughts on living wills. *The Hastings Center Report, 21*, 6–9.

Ross, W. D. (1930). *The right and the good.* New York: Oxford University Press.

Sabatino, C. P. (1993). Surely the wizard will help us too? Implementing the Patient Self-Determination Act. *Hastings Center Report 23*, 12–16.

Sachs, G. A., Stocking, C. E., Miles, S. H. (1992). Failure of an intervention to promote discussion of advance directives. *Journal of the American Geriatrics Society, 40*, 269–73.

Schneiderman, L. J., Kronick, R., Kaplan, R. M., Anderson, J. P., & Langer, R. D. (1992). Effects of offering advance directives on medical treatments and costs. *Annals of Internal Medicine, 117*, 599–606.

Sehgal, A., Galbraith, A., Chesney, M., Schoenfeld, P., Charles, G., & Lo, B. (1992). How strictly do dialysis patients want their advance directives followed? *Journal of the American Medical Association, 267*, 59–63.

Tarnowski, K. J., Allen, D. M., Mayhall, C., & Kelly, P. A. (1990). Readability of pediatric biomedical research informed consent forms. *Pediatrics, 85*, 58–62.

Young, A., Pignatello, C. H., & Taylor, M. B. (1988). Who's the boss? Ethical conflicts in home care. *Health Progress, 69*, 59–62.

Problems and Protocols for Dying at Home in a High-Tech Environment

5

Marshall B. Kapp, J.D., M.P.H.

INTRODUCTION

People were expected to die at home 30 or 40 years ago, and few members of the public or the health professions gave that natural phenomenon much of a second thought. As the technological capabilities of modern medicine have advanced marvelously in our lifetimes,[1] however, the locus of life's ending has changed for many. In its friend of the court brief to the United States Supreme Court in the 1990 *Cruzan*[2] case, the American Hospital Association estimated that 80% of all deaths in this country now take place within the walls of health care institutions. Understandably, most of the legal and ethical analysis of end-of-life issues has therefore been focused on the hospital and, to a much lesser extent, on nursing homes.

Ironically, though, we are beginning to come full circle. Home care is no longer simply custodial in character. Modern technological capabilities enable us to medically treat many patients in the home setting who previously would have needed to receive such treatment (if any were desired) in the acute care hospital.[3] At the same time, an increasing

85

number of people wish to, and believe they can, exercise personal control over the application of that technology better in the home setting than they could as inpatients in a health care institution. As the President's Commission for the Study of Ethical Problems in Medicine noted, "[Because m]any people wish to die at home in familiar surroundings [a]nd, in many cases, hospitals discharge terminally or irreversibly ill patients . . . medical care in the home, especially for terminally and irreversibly ill patients, is increasing."[4]

The advent of high-tech home care for the dying raises a variety of special ethical and legal concerns, as the home environment moves from a place where treatment decisions made elsewhere merely are carried out to a site where decisionmaking itself happens. A search for guidance with these questions in the existing professional literature and case law yields very modest returns, and most of the scant discussion that one does find appears in the nursing, rather than the medical, legal, or ethical publications. There are several possible explanations for this analytic deficit, especially as compared with the cascade of words that have poured forth concerning end-of-life scenarios taking place within institutions.

First, legal and ethical implications of high-tech home care as a setting for dying constitutes a rather new area of study, and therefore simply has been relatively undiscovered by the bioethics community. Second, for most discharge planners, case managers, professional caregivers, patients, and families, the most significant problem relating to home care is an insufficiency of desired and appropriate resources, rather than the spectre of overtreatment at home. The energies of the parties have been concentrated mainly on marshalling adequate resources to satisfy the patient's wants and needs, i.e., the problem of too little, rather than on worrying at length about the problem of too much.[5]

Additionally, comparatively little attention has been devoted to this arena so far perhaps because most judicial decisions and scholarly commentary regarding "death with dignity" or "the right to die" tend to focus on the substantive decisionmaking rights of the parties. In this context it has been automatically taken for granted that home care patients are entitled to the same constitutional and common law protections of autonomy, exercised either directly or through a surrogate applying substituted judgment or best interests standards, as are institutionalized patients. In the leading life-sustaining medical treatment case set in the patient's own home, the New Jersey Supreme Court in 1987 stated categorically that a patient's "right to exercise his or her choice to refuse life-sustaining treatment does not vary depending on whether the patient is in a medical institution or at home."[6] In its 1992 *Guidelines for the Medical Management of the Home Care Patient*, the American Medical Association affirms the right of a home care patient to give or withhold informed consent to any proposed medical treatment.[7]

Even if we accept the proposition that substantive decisional rights are unaffected by the locus of the patient, the practical implementation of those rights raises special ethical and legal wrinkles when the process of dying occurs at home. The issues implicated in the orchestration of a home death are the subject of this chapter, which is intended to ask more questions than it answers. These issues are identified and analyzed through the presentation of several hypothetical cases, set out in what the author judges to be an ascending order of controversy.

CASE

Mr. Jones is a 70-year-old male who has been a heavy smoker for most of his life and has advanced lung cancer, diagnosed a year ago, with a current life expectancy of a few months at most. He is fully cognitive and emotionally capable of making decisions about his medical treatment, and has not been adjudicated otherwise. His physicians have communicated clearly and honestly with him during the course of his disease. Mr. Jones is a widower whose wife died of cancer 4 years ago, and he had lived alone in his own apartment until his last episode of hospitalization for complications of his cancer. Upon discharge, he moved into the home of his daughter (who is his only child) and son-in-law, who have a 17-year-old daughter and a 15-year-old son living at home. Mr. Jones' daughter does not work outside the home, and she and the other family members provide Mr. Jones with substantial informal caregiving.

Mr. Jones receives a substantial monthly pension check based on his many years of work as a university professor, and he is eligible for Medicare. Arrangements have been made for the Acme Home Health Agency, a private, not-for-profit, Medicare-certified organization, to come into the home to provide appropriate health-related services to Mr. Jones on a daily basis.

Mr. Jones is concerned about the anticipated trajectory of his decline and dying over the next several weeks and months, and wishes to maintain as much control over, and dignity and comfort during, his final days as possible.

Ideally, Mr. Jones will be supported and encouraged to think through and express his preferences regarding the initiation, continuation, withholding, or withdrawal of various life-sustaining medical interventions (in his case, probably mechanical ventilation, cardiopulmonary resuscitation, antibiotics, and artificial nutrition) in a clear and timely manner.

In any setting, the role of the patient's physician and other health care providers in initiating and participating honestly in dialogue concerning present and future treatment values and preferences is essential. The patient's home ought to present an especially nonthreatening and congenial (from the patient's perspective) setting for conducting such a sensitive dialogue.

In an interactive caregiver/patient relationship, various contingencies should be investigated with a decisionally capable patient such as Mr. Jones in a dialogue that proceeds over a period of time, rather than in a discussion that begins and shortly thereafter ends at a single point in time. The AMA's home care *Guidelines* recommend that physicians talk with the patient about his or her "participation in treatment decisions and wishes concerning rehospitalization, resuscitation, and use of various medical technologies."[8] Since Mr. Jones is decisionally capable, his family theoretically should be privy to confidential information and participate in treatment discussions only to the extent that Mr. Jones expressly authorizes. However, since Mr. Jones is living in the home of his family and relying heavily on them for informal caregiving, he probably wants their active participation in treatment discussions; in any event, as a practical matter, he probably could not prevent their involvement in this phase of treatment planning. If the family were supporting Mr. Jones' care financially as well, its claim to participation in treatment decision making would be even stronger ethically and more likely practically.

The home care context underscores the importance of the interdisciplinary team involved in the patient's care plan in assisting the patient and family through what may be an extended series of treatment decisions unfolding over time.[9] Predictably, but quite correctly, the nursing literature puts great emphasis on the function of the home care nurse in helping the patient and family to understand treatment and nontreatment options and consequences and in listening to their concerns during multiple conversations.[10] Nurses and other members of the interdisciplinary team must be prepared to participate effectively in these discussions, including preparation for referring the patient to sources of legal and other advice beyond the nurse's expertise,[11] and the present educational void in this area is discussed later.

The conversations about treatment values and preferences taking place between Mr. Jones, his family, and the interdisciplinary team members should be guided by parameters set by Acme Home Care Agency's written organizational policy and procedures on advance medical directives and medical decisionmaking. As a home care agency that is certified to participate in the Medicare and/or Medicaid government financing programs, Acme falls under the requirements contained in the Patient Self-Determination Act enacted by Congress as part of the 1990 Omnibus Budget Reconciliation Act.[12] While this federal statute and the implementing regulations promulgated by the Department of Health and Human Services[13] are not intended to create new substantive patient rights, they do impose a number of procedural obligations on health care providers. Acme is commanded, as a condition of receiving federal dollars for the services it provides, to:

[M]aintain written policies and procedures concerning advance directives with respect to all adult individuals receiving medical care by or through the provider . . .

Provide written information to such individuals [in advance of the individual coming under the care of the agency] concerning—

An individual's rights under State law (whether statutory or recognized by the courts of the State) to make decisions concerning such medical care, including the right to accept or refuse medical or surgical treatment and the right to formulate, at the individual's option, advance directives; and

The written policies of the provider or organization respecting the implementation of such rights, including a clear and precise statement of limitation if the provider cannot implement an advance directive on the basis of conscience;

Document in the individual's medical record whether or not the individual has executed the implementation of such rights [i.e., whether the individual has already made out an advance directive];

Not condition the provision of care or otherwise discriminate against an individual based on whether or not the individual has executed an advance directive;

Ensure compliance with requirements of State law (whether statutory or recognized by the courts of the State) regarding advance directives;

Provide for education of staff concerning its policies and procedures on advance directives; and

Provide for community education to include community

education regarding advance directives . . . , either directly or in concert with other providers and organizations.

Under the same law, each state must,

acting through a State agency, association, or other private nonprofit entity, develop a written description of the State law (whether statutory or as recognized by the courts of the State) concerning advance directives . . . to be distributed by . . . providers . . . in accordance with the requirements [imposed on providers under the Patient Self-Determination Act].[14]

The chief intent of the Act is to enhance patient autonomy by facilitating and encouraging more informed, timely medical decisionmaking, both in terms of the patient's initial selection of a particular provider and of the patient's control regarding specific treatments once the provider/patient relationship has been established. (Success in the practical implementation of the first goal remains to be studied, since it presumes a higher level of opportunity for timely, quality consumer choice among competing providers than the facts may support.) In light of the spirit of the Act, even home health agencies that are not legally bound to do so (that is, even those providers that do not participate in Medicare or Medicaid) ought ethically to create and share with prospective patients formal organizational policies and procedures regarding medical decisionmaking.[15] Besides serving the interests of patient autonomy and informed decisionmaking, notifying the patient and family prospectively of organizational attitudes, particularly concerning any misgivings about honoring patient or family instructions, and internal dispute resolution procedures should proactively help to avoid or mitigate later disagreements about or disruptions in the delivery of care, and certainly should reduce the likelihood of disputes being submitted to the courts for resolution.

The imposition of Patient Self-Determination Act responsibilities on home care providers has not occurred totally without controversy. Some home health agencies have objected to being thrust into an informational role that rightly belongs to the physician as an integral aspect of the physician/patient therapeutic relationship, especially since the physician is the one legally empowered to write the treatment or nontreatment orders for the patient that the home care staff is bound to follow.[16] Some physicians, perhaps jealous of their domain, have joined in this criticism. The problem is that many individuals do not have an established, ongoing relationship with a specific primary care physician, and even those who enjoy such a relationship may find the physician reluctant to participate in, let alone to initiate, conversation about end-of-life treatment issues, especially well before the time that those issues are directly confronting that particular patient. The proper response to this criticism of the Patient Self-Determination Act is not to reduce the informational responsibilities of home care agencies, but rather to encourage physicians to take the initiative in this arena within their medical practices. Physicians should influence general health care policy so that every person enjoys an ongoing primary care physician/patient relationship, within which meaningful discussions about future treatment preferences and values can take place in advance of crisis.

Additionally, the home care agency's formal policies and procedures should explicitly deal with its relationship with the physicians who attend the agency's patients, defining precisely the respective duties and expectations of the parties.[17] Formal concurrence with the agency's policies by the attending physician should be made a condition of affiliation with the agency or, if the patient's right to select a personal physician is considered paramount, the patient should at least be informed early of any serious differences in basic attitudes toward advance directives between agency and physician. Similarly, the home care agency should have policy provisions regarding, and memoranda of understandings with, other relevant independent contractors who may be involved with patient care and with questions of life-sustaining technology usage.

Another somewhat related problem noted with the Patient Self-Determination Act[18] is the proliferation of inconsistent organizational policies and procedures that a single home care patient may encounter. Within the continuum of care that many patients and families experience, they may be exposed to an array of hospitals, nursing homes, and home health agencies, each provider with its own set of policies and procedures concerning medical decisionmaking. Patients and families may receive, and become confused and frustrated by, differing and mixed philosophical signals. The problem can be exacerbated if the patient has recently received medical attention in multiple states. It is conceivable that patients and families caught at a very vulnerable moment, when a patient enters into a home care program from which they are not expected to leave alive, may feel intimidated into executing poorly understood or tepidly embraced advance directives as a result of the cumulative, persuasive effect of confusing but powerful information from different directions.

The federal Patient Self-Determination Act represents just one piece of the intricate legal/regulatory context within which Acme Home Care Agency and Mr. Jones and his family must wend their way toward an acceptable dying scenario.[19] As noted in the earlier discussion of obligations under the Act, each state, as a condition of participation in the Medicaid program, must develop and make available to covered health care providers a written statement of state legislative and judicial policy regarding advance directives and medical decisionmaking. Although certain important ethical principles (such as the right of a currently mentally capable, informed patient like Mr. Jones to voluntarily permit or refuse life-sustaining medical interventions) are by now well entrenched in our national jurisprudence, confusing and restrictive legal vagaries in other details may exist among different states or even within a single state.

Another part of the regulatory atmosphere surrounding

the case of Mr. Jones, and aimed at assuring a minimally acceptable quality of services, consists of pertinent state licensure statutes. (A whole other array of requirements concerning antifraud and abuse, antitrust, and price discrimination regulate the business practices of home care agencies, but these regulations are unlikely to have a significant influence on the process of dying at home,[20] and therefore are not analyzed here.) Mandatory licensure to operate occurs at the level of the home care agency in practically every state, primarily regulating the structural and operational components of the agency.

State licensure also exists at the level of the individual professional staff member who works for the home care agency. Every jurisdiction has professional licensure statutes that restrict the performance of certain services to those individuals who, based upon demonstration of specified education, training, and knowledge, have been licensed by the state to perform those services. Licensure statutes are exclusive or monopolistic, in the sense that unlicensed personnel ordinarily are not legally permitted to perform services that are restricted to licensed professionals. The public policy rationale for these licensure statutes is the inherent state police power, that is, the inherent authority of society to take action to protect and promote the general health, safety, and welfare of the community.

In the home care context, the professional licensure laws of greatest immediate importance are those relating to physicians, nurses, and various forms of therapists (e.g., physical and occupational). The significance of such laws for the topic of this chapter lies in the general rule that, technically speaking, unless a specific exception is present, a family member may not be assigned to perform an activity that is restricted by law to specified licensed professionals (unless, of course, the family member happens to be a licensed member of the relevant profession.)[21] The specific exception to this rule will be discussed below.

For home care agencies (and the majority fall in this category) that are certified for participation in the Medicare program, compliance with the Conditions of Participation set out in 1987 Omnibus Budget Reconciliation Act (OBRA) amendments[22] and implementing regulations[23] are mandatory. Patients' rights provisions of the Conditions of Participation support the concept of patient autonomy and the right to make informed treatment choices.[24]

Home care agencies may seek voluntary accreditation from private accrediting bodies as a visible stamp of approval for their quality of care. The incentive for pursuing such voluntary accreditation has increased recently with the federal government's grant of "deemed status" for Medicare purposes (i.e., acceptance of voluntary accreditation as proof that Medicare standards are being satisfied) to the Community Health Accreditation Program (CHAP) of the National League for Nursing (NLN)[25] and the Joint Commission on Accreditation of Healthcare Organizations (JCAHO).[26] Accreditation standards of these bodies stress the right of informed decisionmaking by patients and the duty of home care agencies to implement procedures for promoting patient autonomy.[27] Additionally, the major trade association in this arena, the National Association for Home Care (NAHC),[28] wrote a provision into its 1989 Model Home Care Bill of Rights respecting the patient's right to refuse specific services. The provision retains the agency's prerogative to refer a patient to another provider, or back to the patient's personal physician, if the patient's refusal to comply with a recommended plan of care compromises the agency's commitment to quality care. Most states have conscience clauses in their advance directive statutes (discussed below) allowing noncompliance with patient treatment wishes based on the provider's philosophical disagreement, as long as the patient has been informed beforehand of this contingency. Presumably, these conscience clauses would apply as well to philosophical disagreements with a currently decisonally capable patient.

The statutes against elder abuse and neglect that have been enacted in every jurisdiction over the past two decades may lead to criminal and/or civil sanctions against home care agencies for the acts and omissions of staff.[29] Ronald Bayer has warned,

> If we decentralize the care of the elderly and frail, the possibility of hidden neglect will increase. It will be very difficult to monitor what goes on behind those millions of closed doors. This is the first and pre-eminent risk associated with the home care movement: Neglect masquerading as more humane care.[30]

State abuse and neglect statutes are not intended to inhibit Acme Home Care Agency from respecting and supporting the choice of Mr. Jones and his family to forego aggressive medical intervention in the final days in favor of palliative care. It is conceivable, though quite unlikely, that some outside organization or individual might complain to a law enforcement entity about the situation. While negative repercussions for the family or Acme would be extremely speculative, even their remote spectre and the negative accompanying publicity could act as an inhibiting factor for certain unduly nervous families and home care agencies.

The free-floating anxiety about potential malpractice lawsuits that pervades the health care industry today cannot be overlooked in any discussion of the delivery of health-related patient services. In addition to the systemic barriers that limit the bringing of malpractice actions against professional providers in the home care arena generally,[31] Acme's conscientious inclusion of Mr. Jones' family in discussions about Mr. Jones' treatment choices, its compliance with its own written policies and procedures regarding medical decisionmaking, and its careful documentation of all communications and actions constitute a sensible risk management strategy that should assure that malpractice fears do not interfere with ethical conduct in this case.

It has been suggested that the presence of these various quality assurance mechanisms, plus the fact that few home care agencies have yet developed formal, permanent inter-

nal mechanisms for assisting with the handling of bioethi-
cal issues, may lead to more external scrutiny of private
agreements to abate certain life-sustaining medical interventions in the home setting. At the same time, others have
speculated that professionals may fail to probe and push a
patient's treatment refusal as hard in the home environment as they would in a hospital or nursing home, and that
providers may be more likely to accept the home care patient's purported decision to limit life-sustaining medical
interventions at face value.[32] This may be especially objectionable if the patient's decision to forego life-sustaining
treatments is less than truly informed or capable, because
the patient underestimated and underappreciated the risks
and consequences involved, reasoning erroneously that "If
I were really sick, I would be in a hospital. I must be all
right if I'm at home."[33]

Dubler has argued that the presumption in favor of a patient's right to make such decisions ought to be stronger in
the home care than the institutional setting.[34] In judging decisional capacity, she urges, the authenticity of the patient's choice should be afforded more weight than the
present cognitive ability to manipulate factual information
and deliberate rationally. Indeed, the natural, familiar, and
nonthreatening surroundings of home should enhance both
the patient's cognitive capacities and the ability to make decisions consistent with previously held values and preferences, thereby justifying deference to the patient's spoken
choice. Further, Dubler has pointed to the difficulty of conducting many sophisticated diagnostic tests in the patient's
home, thereby decreasing the degree of medical certainty
with which expected benefits of treatment may be predicted, and hence diminishing the authority attaching to
any recommendations in favor of aggressive interventions
entailing life-sustaining medical technologies.[35]

Against the foregoing background, what is the proper
role for Mr. Jones' family regarding, first, the process of decisionmaking about various life-sustaining medical interventions for Mr. Jones and, second, informal caregiving and

support for Mr. Jones in implementing whatever treatment decisions are made?

Theoretically, for a decisionally capable patient like Mr. Jones, the family's role would consist solely of, first, advising Mr. Jones to the extent that he requested, as he rationally evaluated information communicated to him by the interdisciplinary home care team in the light of his lifetime of accummulated values and preferences and, second, supporting him in fulfilling his choice. More commonly, medical decisionmaking at home will probably be a joint or shared endeavor,[36] with the family either giving support to or placing pressure on the patient in either direction. When the patient and home care providers disagree about the wisdom of specific treatments, families can make it easier or harder for the professionals to "gang up" on the patient.[37] When a disagreement exists between even a decisionally capable patient and the family (or some of its members), family interests in determining the outcome arguably take on ethical significance in direct proportion to the degree that the family will be involved in paying for and/or personally providing the care necessary to effectuate the choices reached.[38]

Therein lies the crux of the family's role. Mr. Jones retains what Collopy has described as decisional autonomy, but lacks its executional counterpart.[39] Put differently, Mr. Jones may have the right to make his own choices about medical treatment, but he must depend heavily on his family to care for him as an essential part of the fulfillment of his decisions.

The hypothetical case of Mr. Jones has been crafted to approximate the ideal "Rockwellian image of high tech/ high touch," described by one author as "the trigenerational family sitting by the hearth with a back-up oxygen tank perched next to the grandfather clock."[40] One need not subscribe to former Vice-President Quayle's sociological interpretation of the modern American family to believe that, for most real families, the family/patient relationship engendered by the experience of informal caregiving will be considerably more complex and difficult.

Feinberg has written:

> The assumptions of high tech home care can be perceived as an assault on the independence and autonomy of the middle-aged adult child of elderly parents. It reverses the pattern of decreasing dependence that is a hallmark of the evolving family system and demands a return to a concept of the original nuclear family as deeply interconnected for the duration of the life of the last surviving parent. High tech home care raises fundamental ethical questions regarding the nature of family relationships [and] the priorities of obligation . . .[41]

In assessing what the family owes[42] to its dependent members, we should consider the material and human costs in terms of lost income, leisure and career opportunities, and interaction with other family members.

From a legal perspective, over half the states have statutes on the books that impose some financial obligation on adult children for the long-term care of indigent parents, although enforcement efforts usually are anemic. No state imposes, or could impose, a binding duty on an adult child to actually deliver caregiver services personally to a parent.[43]

As alluded to earlier, professional licensure laws may act as a complicating factor concerning informal caregiving by families. Where willing and able family members are available, it is typical for home care agencies to train those individuals to provide certain personal care and homemaker services for the patient. Concerning health-related services, most state Nurse Practice Acts explicitly exempt from their restrictions services provided by family (and in most cases friends also) to relatives in their own homes. Research reveals no reported findings of liability against either a family member or a supervising home care agency for negligence by the family member in the performance of health-related services within the patient's home.

Mr. Jones may require various medications over the next few weeks or months in order to die comfortably and peacefully at home. No state explicitly empowers family members to administer medications; neither do most states expressly prohibit family from doing so. It is generally accepted that family members may help the patient to take over-the-counter medications (e.g., by opening, holding, or even emptying medicine containers). The ability of family members to administer prescription drugs without technically violating Nurse Practice Acts is more problematic. As a practical matter, however, relatives do help home care patients take medications thousands of times a day around the country without any reported prosecutions for practicing nursing without a license. The picture becomes cloudier still in questioning whether other health-related tasks may be delegated to family members. Again, there is a dearth of reported case law on this subject. Home care agencies thus far have proceeded in the delegation of tasks to family members with a minimum of anxiety for liability associated with acts and omissions of those individuals, and this attitude is borne out by practical experience. At least 23 states, in their exemptions to the Nurse Practice Act, expressly require that home care services by family members or friends be provided gratuitously, while other states are silent on the question of compensating relatives.

When caregiving tasks have been taken on by the family, a question may arise about the ethical and legal authority, or conversely the responsibility, to intervene when the family is failing in those tasks to the patient's detriment. It is very unclear at what point, if any, the home care agency would be compelled to cease looking the other way and take action as the patient's advocate, either morally or under mandate of the state's adult abuse and neglect reporting statute.[44]

CASE

In the second hypothetical case, Mr. Jones is severely decisionally incapacitated at the time of his last hospital discharge, although he has not been adjudicated incompetent by a probate court. However, 6 months earlier, while he was still decisionally capable, Mr. Jones had visited an attorney with his daughter and executed both an instruction directive, stating that no "heroic measures" should be utilized to keep him alive artificially after there was no hope of recovery, and a proxy directive, naming the daughter as his surrogate decisionmaking agent in the event of his future incapacity.

In this case, Mr. Jones' advance directives would be useful in determining his future, and final, course of care at home.[45] Legislation has now been enacted in every state describing the process for executing such directives. State "Natural Death" laws authorize both living wills or declarations (instruction directives) and durable powers of attorney for health care (proxy directives). Some confusion may arise over the particular interpretation of some state statutes that, read on their face, appear to restrict the prerogatives of decisionally capable individuals to direct future treatment in certain respects. The better view is that state legislation may only procedurally effectuate or substantively expand, but may not substantively limit, the constitutional decisional rights that have been recognized in the medical treatment area.[46]

One may find successful experiences with the use of advance medical directives in the home care setting. One pilot project[47] involved an initial approach by the physician to the home care patient about the opportunity to execute a durable power of attorney, followed by an attempt to have the named agent, if any, present at the next physician/patient home encounter. If the named proxy could not attend the next home care appointment, the patient was instructed to at least discuss treatment values and preferences personally with the proxy as soon as possible. The project's emphasis on proxy decisionmakers may have been less intimidating, and hence more readily accepted by patients, than confronting the patient directly with decisions about withholding or withdrawing life-sustaining technological interventions. The study found, consistent with the experience of other home care programs,[48] that most home care patients welcomed these discussions, and extremely few found them upsetting. When patients later became decisionally incapacitated and seriously ill, both physicians and proxies found their previous discussions with the patient quite helpful in understanding the patient's point of view. The proxy was more likely to understand, respect, and honor the patient's wishes, especially where the proxy had witnessed or participated in a physician/patient interchange about treatment preferences.

Another form of advance or prospective medical directive that might follow from Mr. Jones' living will, from conversations with the named agent under the durable power of attorney, or from earlier conversations between a previously decisionally capable Mr. Jones and the home health team, would be orders written by Mr. Jones' physician to other health care providers to refrain from initiating particular interventions. These "Do Not" orders might involve hospitalization, intubation, or a variety of other potential interventions that Mr. Jones previously indicated a desire to avoid under certain circumstances. Most ethical and legal attention to "Do Not" orders thus far, though, has revolved around cardiopulmonary resuscitation (CPR) (using CPR here as shorthand for an array of basic and advanced cardiac life support technologies).[49]

As a general proposition, there is a strong legal and ethical presumption in favor of the initiation of CPR for a patient who has suffered a cardiac arrest. This presumption would be overcome, however, in this second Mr. Jones case. Mr. Jones, while still decisionally capable, had made a decision, informed by his conversations with the health care team and supported by his family, to forego CPR in the event of arrest because the anticipated physical, psychological, and financial burdens to Mr. Jones would outweigh the minimal expected benefit of, at most, a short life extension with poor quality until the next arrest.

Reports of home care programs' experience in conducting Do Not Resuscitate (DNR) discussions reveal that few patients or families are reluctant to engage in the conversation, and most are thankful when the subject is broached. Among the benefits of these homebased conversations noted are:

1) an opportunity for the physician and other members of the interdisciplinary team to review with the patient and family the patient's condition and prognosis;

2) letting the patient maintain more control and involvement in the discussion than would probably occur in an inpatient environment;

3) having families hear, and therefore later be more likely to accept, the patient's wishes as expressed in a friendly, familiar atmosphere;

4) in a situation where the patient enters a hospital, for instance to address a treatable intercurrent illness, equipping the home care physician to talk knowledgeably to house staff and attending physicians about the patient's preferences; and

5) priming the patient, with or without a DNR order, for subsequent discussions if his or her medical status deteriorates further.[50]

A problem might occur if, upon Mr. Jones' cardiac arrest at home, his family panicked and called the emergency rescue squad instead of passively watching Mr. Jones die. This is a common scenario.[51] When this happens, it is standard practice for the emergency squad arriving at the home to be guided by the normal presumption in favor of rescue intervention and to override any family protestations at that point to let the patient die peacefully.[52]

In an attempt to address this problem and to assure that home care patient wishes regarding the withholding of CPR are honored, emergency medical personnel and other pertinent components of the health care system (e.g., medical societies, hospital and nursing home associations, home care agencies, and hospices) in a growing number of states and

localities are working jointly to establish formal prehospital or "portable" DNR policies and procedures to confer legal protection on emergency squads for respecting home-
based CPR orders while guarding against mistakes that
could jeopardize patients who want every last ounce of
medical technology.[53] The content of these policies and procedures varies widely in terms of medical interventions
that may be covered by a prehospital "Do Not" order and
the means of documenting and validating the order to withhold.[54] As of 1993, 17 states (AR, AZ, CO, FL, IL, MD, MT,
NM, NY, PA, RI, TN, UT, VA, WY, WA, WV) had passed legislation authorizing out-of-hospital DNR orders. One set of
authors has suggested that, for withholding CPR at home,
specific physician-written DNR orders are preferable to relying exclusively on more global instruction directives, because the latter requires too much interpretation for the
emergency medical services context.[55]

The American College of Emergency Physicians has published *Guidelines for Do Not Resuscitate Orders in the Prehospital Setting*.[56] This document is intended to provide procedural assistance only, and not to affect criteria for
decisionmaking itself.

Many administrative barriers impede the progress of implementing prehospital "Do Not" orders in a number of localities. There are logistical questions regarding the form
and timeliness of documentation and procedures for au-
thenticating orders, as well as the energy necessary to re-
educate and coordinate numerous interacting players (e.g.,
patients and families, local governments sponsoring emergency squads and the agencies operating them, physicians,
and home care personnel) who may be ignorant of the issues and engaged in petty but powerful turf battles.[57]

Fear of legal liability can be a serious impediment, especially where attorneys with no health law or bioethics background are counselling local municipalities clients who operate emergency medical squads with unreasonable and
ill-informed advice to continue resuscitating every home care
patient for whom they are called, regardless of physician or-

ders to the contrary. Although special immunity statutes are not legally necessary to protect emergency medical personnel who honor a properly executed home-based DNR order, such legislation unfortunately may be required psychologically to encourage desired behaviors. The Colorado Department of Health, for example, in 1992 promulgated rules, protocols, and sample forms pertaining to implementation of advance medical directives for CPR by emergency medical service personnel under the authority of recent legislation specifically enacted for that purpose.[58]

In this second hypothetical case, where a presently incapacitated Mr. Jones previously executed advance directives while still decisionally capable, the family's role is central in fulfilling Mr. Jones' treatment values and preferences. They should support those preferences and help interpret them to members of the home care team. Where specific decisions arise about which Mr. Jones previously expressed no clear preferences, it is up to the family (and especially the daughter, who is designated the agent by the proxy directive) to guide medical conduct according to the principles of substituted judgment (i.e., what Mr. Jones would want if presently able to make and express autonomous, authentic choices) or, if substituted judgment is not realistic, consistent with Mr. Jones' best interests. Finally, the family will need to continue working with the formal home care professionals in providing informal care consistent with Mr. Jones' wishes as long as he lives.

CASE

Mr. Jones has become decisionally incapable and has not previously executed any advance directive or otherwise clearly and consistently indicated his personal values and preferences concerning the initiation, continuation, withholding, or withdrawal of life-sustaining medical interventions for himself near the end of life.

At this point, the role of Mr. Jones' family would become paramount. In the majority of jurisdictions today, Mr.

AUTHORIZED AGENT'S DIRECTIVE TO WITHHOLD CARDIOPULMONARY RESUSCITATION (CPR)
S-A-M-P-L-E

State of Colorado

Patient's Name: _____

Please Type or Print

Agent's Name: _____

DOB: ____/____/____ Sex: [ ] Male [ ] Female Eye Color: _____
                                          Hair Color: _____

Race: [ ] Black, Non-Hispanic   [ ] Hispanic
      [ ] American Indian or Alaskan   [ ] White, Non-Hispanic
      [ ] Asian or Pacific Islander   [ ] Other _____

Name of Hospice Program (If applicable): _____

Attending Physician's Name: _____

Please Type or Print

Address: _____
          Street   City   Zip

Telephone: (_____) _____-_____ Physicians License #: _____

S-A-M-P-L-E

Directive made this _____ day of _____, 199__, pursuant to Colorado Revised Statute 15-18.6-101.

I, _____, am over the age of 18 years and of sound mind and I am the authorized agent of _____, referred to herein as the "patient".

I have been authorized to act on the patient's behalf in the issuance of this directive.

I have been advised that the expected result of executing this directive is the patient's death in the event the patient's heart or breathing stops.

I hereby direct emergency medical services personnel, health care providers, and any other person, to withhold cardiopulmonary resuscitation in the event the patient's heart or breathing stops. I understand that this directive does not apply to other medical interventions for comfort care. If I am admitted to a health care facility this directive shall be implemented as a physicians' order, pending further physicians' orders.

_____   _____
Signature of Authorized Agent   Signature of Attending Physician

FIGURE 5.1 Authorized agent's directive to withhold cardiopulmonary resuscitation (CPR) sample. *Source*: State of Colorado Department of Health, Denver, CO (1991).

**PATIENT DIRECTIVE TO WITHHOLD
CARDIOPULMONARY RESUSCITATION (CPR)**

S-A-M-P-L-E

State of Colorado

Patient's Name: _____
                        Please Type or Print

DOB: ____/____/____ Sex: [ ] Male [ ] Female   Eye Color: _____
                                                 Hair Color: _____

Race: [ ] Black, Non-Hispanic   [ ] Hispanic
       [ ] American Indian or Alaskan [ ] White, Non-Hispanic
       [ ] Asian or Pacific Islander [ ] Other _____

Name of Hospice Program (If applicable): _____

Attending Physician's Name: _____
                                          Type or Print

Address: _____
              Street   City   Zip

Telephone: (____) ____-_____ Physician's License #: _____

S-A-M-P-L-E

Directive made this _____ day of _____, 199__, pursuant to
     Colorado Revised Statute   15-18.6-101.

I, _____, am over the age of 18 years, of sound
     mind, and acting voluntarily.

It is my desire to initiate this directive on my behalf and I have been
     advised that the expected result of executing this directive is my
     death, in the event that my heart or breathing stops.

I hereby direct emergency medical services personnel, health care providers,
     and other persons to withhold cardiopulmonary resuscitation in the event
     that my heart or breathing stops. I understand that this directive does
     not apply to other medical interventions for comfort care. If I am
     admitted to a health care facility this directive shall be implemented
     as a physicians' order, pending further physicians' orders

_____   _____
     Signature of Patient   Signature of Attending Physician

FIGURE 5.2 Patient directive to withhold cardiopulmonary resuscitation (CPR) sample. *Source*: State of Colorado Department of Health, Denver, CO (1991).

Jones' family members, in a stated priority order, would be empowered by state statute to make surrogate medical decisions on behalf of the incapacitated Mr. Jones who created no advance instructions.[59] The specific content of these surrogate decisionmaking statutes varies widely among jurisdictions, both in terms of restrictions on the type of decision allowed and the procedural hurdles erected purportedly to protect the vulnerable patient.[60] Among the decisions that families ordinarily are permitted to make are those pertaining to the type of prospective "Do Not" orders discussed above. The family member(s) acting as surrogate decision maker is expected to make choices consistent either with substituted judgment (to the extent that the patient's own wishes might be inferred from the totality of past statements and conduct) or best interests principles. In some states without this type of legislation, judicial precedent formally legitimizes the family's role.

Even in the absence of authorizing state legislation or precise judicial precedent, the longstanding and broadly accepted medical tradition in this kind of situation has been reliance on family members.[61] This informal practice of looking to "next of kin" has been challenged only by a small minority of commentators, who would require an adversary hearing and judicial approval for every life-sustaining medical treatment withholding or withdrawal decision for a decisionally incapable patient.[62] The unappealing alternatives to informal reliance on next of kin, in the absence of specific state family surrogate consent legislation or judicial precedent legitimizing in advance the family's authority, would be either routine initiation of guardianship proceedings (assuming that an appropriate individual is willing and available to be named guardian by the court) or waiting until a medical emergency has materialized and then providing intervention (likely by transfer to a hospital) based on the emergency exception to informed consent. As a practical matter, as noted by legal counsel for the National Association for Home Care, a home health provider that is unduly obsessed with potential liability and "that insists on a formal authorization for surrogate or substitute decision making may be unable to provide care in any fashion at all."[63]

Mr. Jones' daughter is presumably the most appropriate surrogate decisionmaker in this case[64] because she probably knows her father and his values better than anyone else alive; she is likely to have his best interests at heart, and she will be the one most intimately and directly affected—both as caregiver and eventual mourner—by the consequences of medical decisions made and implemented concerning Mr. Jones. Deference to the family admittedly is not without some dangers, though. In the home environment, families may find their informal caregiving burdens overwhelming, and hence may be overly anxious to bring down the final curtain. Conversely, the family that can go home at night after visiting a relative in a hospital or nursing home may be more willing to insist unreasonably on "Doing Everything," since its members do not have to live quite as intensely and unrelentingly in the middle of the drama.

Professional home caregivers certainly must be sensitive to potential emotional or financial conflicts of interest between the family and a decisionally incapable, vulnerable patient. The possibility of such a conflict, though, should not negate the usual presumption in favor of the family acting as decisional surrogate for Mr. Jones.

Let us assume that Mr. Jones' family, based on their educated surmise about what Mr. Jones would want or on their assessment of his best interests in light of the balance between likely burdens and benefits, decides to maintain Mr. Jones in their home to die without the initiation of high-tech life-sustaining medical interventions. The family may still agree to hospitalization and limited treatment for intercurrent illness (e.g., a broken leg, breathing difficulties, or tooth abscess) that can fairly easily be reversed and whose reversal would materially improve the patient's comfort and enjoyment during whatever life remains.[65] Following the limited treatment, the patient may be returned from the hospital to continue with the plan to die at home in peace and comfort.

CASE

In the fourth hypothetical situation, Mr. Jones presently is decisionally capable and, fearing a long, difficult physical and mental decline that will be painful for him and burdensome for his family, asks his physician to provide the means (e.g., a large number of sedatives) by which Mr. Jones can at any time terminate his own life.

A similar fact pattern emerged in the case of young adult quadriplegic Larry McAfee. The Georgia Supreme Court held that the patient possessed a constitutional right to control a switch that had been devised for him that would permanently shut off the ventilator upon which he was dependent for life. The court also held that any health professional who gave Mr. McAfee pain medications so that he could die peacefully once the ventilator were withdrawn would be immune from liability, although no professional could be forced to participate.[66]

The ethical and legal implications of physician-assisted suicide have been much in the news lately, and a rehearsal of these issues is beyond the scope of this chapter. Suffice it to note that the home environment's relative sheltering from the extensive external oversight that characterizes modern health care institutions makes it a likely site for the expansion of various forms of assisted suicide that are acknowledged to happen but without being labelled as such. The family's complicity in assisted suicide schemes, although theoretically irrelevant because the patient is decisionally capable and physically able to carry out the decisive act, in reality is indispensable. The family caring for Mr. Jones at home is in a position to thwart his assisted suicide attempt (e.g., by taking away his lethal supply of pills or calling the emergency squad and demanding resuscitation) or to facilitate it (e.g., by getting the presescription filled and opening the bottle).

CASE

A decisionally capable Mr. Jones, in this hypothetical circumstance, asks his physician, perhaps in conjunction with
other members of the interdisciplinary team, to come to his
daughter's home where he is living and to give him a lethal
injection to "put him out of his misery."

What Mr. Jones is requesting is active euthanasia, which
is illegal in every American jurisdiction. The ethical and
public policy ramifications of active euthanasia have drawn
heavy commentary recently, and full explorations may be
found elsewhere. Suffice it to note here, as with the previous hypothetical case, that home care may provide a relatively sheltered setting in which controversial practices are
less likely to be detected, questioned, and punished—and
therefore are more likely to occur—than would be true in a
health care institutional environment. Here, too, the ability
of the health care team to carry out Mr. Jones' expressed
wish would, practically speaking, be impossible without
the complicity and cooperation of his family. Indeed, the involvement of the health care team may not even be necessary; the family could, for instance, purposely turn off a
ventilator and blame the death on equipment failure or accident[67] (although many would categorize this as passive,
rather than active, euthanasia).

CASE

In the final scenario, the professional home care providers
and the family agree that active or involuntary euthanasia
should be performed upon a decisionally incapacitated Mr.
Jones.

The law, and most current ethical thinking, would con-
demn action, such as a lethal injection administered for the
purpose and with the intent of hastening Mr. Jones' death.
On the other hand, some action, such as the family detach-
ing a ventilator, would be easier to justify as passive rather

than active conduct; much less likely to come to the attention of law enforcement personnel; and extremely unlikely to be punished if it were detected.

POST-DEATH ISSUES

After Mr. Jones has died, several things ordinarily or potentially would occur that have legal and ethical ramifications. Foresight about these post-death events might affect the way in which the death itself is orchestrated at home.

In every state, upon a patient's death the attending physician usually is responsible for filling out the medical portion of the death certificate. In certain circumstances, the attending physician is required by statute to report the circumstances of a patient's death (regardless of where it occurs) to a local public official, either a coroner or a medical examiner, depending on the public death investigation system in place in the particular jurisdiction. This public official then determines what steps, if any, including an autopsy, are appropriate to investigate the deceased's death. When a case is within the jurisdiction of the coroner or medical examiner, the deceased's family may not prevent a public investigation from proceeding; the family's consent for autopsy or other measures is not legally necessary.

State statutes differ in detail concerning when an attending physician is mandated to report a patient's death to the coroner or medical examiner. Standard grounds for mandatory death reporting include the following:

a) There is a reasonable belief of criminal activity;
b) there is a reasonable belief that the death was violent in nature;
c) the death occurred by casualty (accident);
d) the death was an apparent suicide;
e) the individual died suddenly when in apparent good health; and

f) the death occurred in any suspicious or unusual manner.

Once a coroner or medical examiner has conducted an autopsy, some states treat the results as an easily accessible public document, whereas other states prevent the public from obtaining the resulting information.

These reporting and investigation requirements introduce an element of potential retrospective oversight that may influence the willingness of physicians and other home care providers to implement certain treatment decisions, such as those involving active euthanasia via a mechanism like lethal injection. It is conceivable, though, that in the home care setting certain technological and documentation strategies are easier to employ to reduce the legal risks associated with retrospective review of potentially controversial behavior than would be the case in a health care institution.

Ideally, Acme Home Care Agency will have made prior arrangements with Mr. Jones' attending physician, the local coroner, and the funeral director regarding pronouncement of death and disposition of the deceased's body.[68] Some families, such as those wishing to verify a diagnosis of Alzheimer's disease, might voluntarily make arrangements at this point for a partial or complete autopsy. The patient, while decisionally capable, may have left permission for autopsy (e.g., for educational purposes), and arrangements must be made for carrying out this last wish. Acme should have written policies and procedures detailing how these arrangements will be handled, and the specifics should be discussed ahead of time with Mr. Jones (if capable of participating) and his family.

Prior arrangements ideally also will be made regarding procurement of organs from the deceased that he or she previously was, or that the family currently is, willing to donate for transplantation purposes. It is unlikely that Mr. Jones would have viable transplantable organs, but some patients who die planned deaths at home will have usable

organs. Acme should have a written policy on the organ donation and harvesting issue.

PUBLIC POLICY RECOMMENDATIONS

The trend toward more seriously ill Americans living and
dying at home is a positive one, even if some of the underlying reasons for this trend are disturbing. If the home-based
death phenomenon is to continue, flourish, and accomplish
the objective of assuring peaceful, dignified, and autonomous final days, some of the present legal and ethical ambi-
guity infusing the subject must be addressed. This chapter
offers a very tentative and abbreviated list of possible public policy initiatives aimed in this direction.

First, states should relax and/or clarify regulatory restrictions, particularly those in Nurse Practice Acts, concerning the permissible role of families in providing health-
related home services. Such a move could significantly
enhance salutary family involvement in supporting the patient at the end of life.

Second, states should consider (as a few already have)
amending their statutes to permit nonphysicians (namely,
nurses) to declare death under certain carefully delineated
circumstances, such as where an expected home-based
death occurs and the nurse has been certified as qualified
to do this. Alternatively (e.g., Ohio), state law could continue to require that physicians declare death, but permit
the declaration to occur based on facts supplied to the physician by another health professional. Requiring that a physician physically appear at the home to pronounce the obvious often results in unnecessary delay, inconvenience, and
stress for all involved.

Third, a massive educational campaign is overdue. The
general public, including potential patients and their families and physicians, must be better informed about medical
options in the home care setting, the proper use of emergency medical systems, and the surrounding ethical and le-

gal issues. Home care professionals must be better prepared to provide timely, accurate information and counsel
to those they serve.[69] The Home Health Assembly of New
Jersey has developed a good prototype of an educational
strategy for informing home health agencies and their personnel about pertinent ethical topics.[70]

Fourth, home health agencies, acting singly or through
consortia arrangements, need to develop ethics committees
or their equivalents to help on an ongoing basis with education, policy development and implementation, and individual concurrent or retrospective case consultation concerning recurring ethical and legal questions.[71] Ethics
committees can legitimize the importance of ethical practice, provide a conducive milieu for problem solving, and
establish an intellectual framework for engaging in the decisionmaking process. Special selling points for some form
of ethics committee in home care include the changing nature of the home care enterprise because of technology development and rising concern about escalating costs; home
care workers who often act independently without much
oversight or supervision and thus are thrust into "tight"
ethical and legal spots without sufficient support; and the
present lack of formal ethical preparation that most home
care personel bring to their jobs.[72]

Fifth, the turf battles alluded to earlier must be worked
out. These inhibit the effective development and implementation of prehospital DNR policies and procedures that
would allow panicky families to call emergency squads
without subjecting the arresting patient to unwanted resuscitation attempts or more aggressive medical assaults. Prehospital emergency providers must be educated, as must be
their attorneys and the community physicians who write
orders concerning the limitation of treatment for home-
based patients.

Finally, society must supply a more adequate, accessible
arsenal of resources to support families during the difficult
final period of caring for a dying patient at home. Home
care must not mean an abandonment of the family on

whom the patient happily has been dumped. The tolerance of family members for a relative dying, sometimes quite slowly, at home depends a lot on the support available to them. Is a nurse or physician readily available to come to the home to assess changes in symptoms and to help with emotional and administrative concerns at the time of death? The current organizational and financial structure of the health care system frequently makes this difficult.[73] As Erich Loewy points out, however, support needs are not always tangible. One of the reasons that families panic when even an anticipated cardiac arrest takes place at home is a concern with what the neighbors may think if "help" is not immediately summoned. Home care and its associated emergencies do not occur in a social vacuum, and informal communities (e.g., neighbors, churches, friends) also must be educated to support families caring for dying patients at home.[74] The availability of support groups sponsored by specific disease-oriented associations (e.g., Alzheimer's, multiple sclerosis, muscular dystrophy, AIDS) can also be quite valuable.

CONCLUSION

Dying at home is hard, because it requires the active support of one's family or other living companions and of physicians and other health care professionals for general humanitarian and comfort care during what may be a very slow and draining process. The tension between medical and social models of home care may easily reach a breaking point.[75] How our society resolves and accommodates the ethical and legal questions implicated by the choice to die at home will go far toward defining home care as either a simple change in site for the provision of high-tech medical treatment, or a broader change in the range of choices and services available to dying persons and in our conceptualization of care itself at the end of life.

ACKNOWLEDGMENTS

This chapter is based on a paper originally commissioned by the Montefiore Medical Center Project on *The Technological Tether: Ethical and Social Dimensions of High-Tech Home Care*. A shorter version will appear in a book by that title edited by John Arras and Nancy N. Dubler. This project was sponsored by the Greenwall Foundation and the Commonwealth Fund.

REFERENCES

1. U.S. Congress, Office of Technology Assessment, LIFE-SUSTAINING TECHNOLOGY AND THE ELDERLY. Washington, DC: U.S. Government Printing Office (1987).

2. *Cruzan v. Director, Missouri Department of Health*, 110 S.Ct. 2841 (1990).

3. Knight Steel, "Home Care for the Elderly: The New Institution," 151 ARCHIVES OF INTERNAL MEDICINE 439–442 (March 1991).

4. President's Commission for the Study of Ethical Problems in Medicine and Biomedical and Behavioral Research, DECIDING TO FOREGO LIFE-SUSTAINING TREATMENT. Washington, DC: U.S. Government Printing Office (March 1983), at 103.

5. Reckling, JoAnn B. "Abandonment of Patients by Home Health Nursing Agencies: An Ethical Analysis of the Dilemma," 11(3) ADVANCES IN NURSING SCIENCE 70–81 (1989).

6. *In re Farrell*, 108 N.J. 335, 529 A.2d 404, 413–14 (1987).

7. American Medical Association, Department of Geriatric Health, GUIDELINES FOR MEDICAL MANAGEMENT OF THE HOME CARE PATIENT. Chicago: AMA (1992), at 15.

8. *Id.*, at 6.

9. *Id.*, at 10–14.

10. Beverly R. Bigler, "Critical Care Nursing: Expanding Roles and Responsibilities Within the Community," 2 CRITICAL CARE NURSING CLINICS OF NORTH AMERICA 493–502, 495 (September 1990); Louise M. Brown & G. Kay Rousseau, "Resuscitation

Status Begins at Home," 90 AMERICAN JOURNAL OF NURSING 24 (April 1990).

11. Pat Carr, "Implications of the Implementation of the Patient Self-Determination Act for Nurses in the Field," 10 HOME HEALTHCARE NURSE 53–54 (March-April 1992).

12. Public Law 101–508 (1990), §§ 4206 (Medicare) and 4751 (Medicaid).

13. 42 Code of Federal Regulations §489.102.

14. 42 Code of Federal Regulations §431.20.

15. Marshelle Thobaben, "The Legal and Moral Obligations of Home Care Agencies With Regard to the New Patient Self-Determination Act," 10 HOME HEALTHCARE NURSE 55–56 (March-April 1992).

16. William A. Dombi, "The Patient's Right of Self-Determination," CARING MAGAZINE 78–82 (May 1991).

17. Amy M. Haddad & Marshall B. Kapp, ETHICAL AND LEGAL ISSUES IN HOME HEALTH CARE. Norwalk, CT: Appleton & Lange (1991), at 96.

18. Id.

19. Allen D. Spiegel, "Regulation of High Technology Home Care," in DELIVERING HIGH TECHNOLOGY HOME CARE (Maxwell J. Mehlman & Stuart J. Younger, eds.). New York: Springer Publishing Company (1991), at 67–83.

20. Marshall B. Kapp, GERIATRICS AND THE LAW: PATIENT RIGHTS AND PROFESSIONAL RESPONSIBILITIES, Second Edition. New York: Springer Publishing Company (1992), at 187.

21. Marshall B. Kapp, "Improving Choices Regarding Home Care Services: Legal Impediments and Empowerments," 10 SAINT LOUIS UNIVERSITY PUBLIC LAW REVIEW 441–484, 449–450 (1991).

22. Public Law 100–203, 101 Stat. 1330–67–1330–75, Title IV (Subpart B) (1987).

23. 42 Code of Federal Regulations Part 484. Slightly revised final regulations were published at 56 Federal Register 32967–32975 (July 18, 1991).

24. 42 Code of Federal Regulations §484.10 (c).

25. 57 Federal Register 22273–79 (May 29, 1992).

26. 58 Federal Register 35,007–35,017 (June 30, 1993).

27. Joint Commission on Accreditation of Healthcare Organizations, ACCREDITATION MANUAL FOR HOME CARE, VOLUME 1: HOME CARE STANDARDS. Chicago (1993).

28. National Association for Home Care, Model Home Care Bill of Rights. (1989). Washington, DC: Author.

29. *Caretenders, Inc.* v. *Commonwealth*, Kentucky Court of Appeals (September 21, 1990).

30. Ronald Bayer, "Ethics in Home Care and Quality Assurance," 5(1) CARING 50–56, at 55 (1986).

31. Sandra H, Johnson, "Liability Issues," in DELIVERING HIGH TECHNOLOGY HOME CARE (Maxwell J. Mehlman & Stuart J. Youngner, eds.). New York: Springer Publishing Company (1991), at 125–159.

32. Bart Collopy, Nancy Dubler, & Connie Zuckerman, "The Ethics of Home Care: Autonomy and Accommodation," 20 HASTINGS CENTER REPORT 1–16 (Supplement March/April 1990).

33. *Id.*, at 8.

34. Nancy N. Dubler, "Refusals of Medical Care in the Home Setting," 18 LAW, MEDICINE & HEALTH CARE 227–33, 231 (Fall 1990).

35. *Id.*, at 229.

36. Marshall B. Kapp, "Health Care Decision Making By the Elderly: I Get By With a Little Help From My Family," 31 GERONTOLOGIST 619–623 (October 1991).

37. Dubler, *supra*, note 34, at 229.

38. Nancy N. Dubler, ETHICS ON CALL: A MEDICAL ETHICIST SHOWS HOW TO TAKE CHARGE OF LIFE-AND-DEATH CHOICES. New York: Harmony Books (1992), at 216–222.

39. Bart J. Collopy, "Autonomy in Long Term Care: Some Crucial Distinctions," 28 GERONTOLOGIST 10–17 (Supplement June 1988).

40. Edward A. Feinberg, "Ethical Issues," in DELIVERING HIGH TECHNOLOGY HOME CARE (Maxwell J. Mehlman & Stuart J. Younger, eds.). New York: Springer Publishing Company (1991), at 84–124, 95.

41. *Id.*

42. Daniel Callahan, "What Do Children Owe Elderly Parents?" 15(2) HASTINGS CENTER REPORT 32–37 (1985).

43. Marshall B. Kapp, "Legal and Ethical Issues in Family Caregiving and the Role of Public Policy," 12 HOME HEALTH-CARE SERVICES QUARTERLY 5–28 (1991).

44. Collopy, Dubler, & Zuckerman, *supra* note 32, at 11.

45. Nancy I. Connaway, "Relying on the Living Will in Home Health Care," 3 HOME HEALTHCARE NURSE 42–45 (March-April 1985).

46. Marshall B. Kapp, "State Statutes Limiting Advance Directives: Death Warrants or Life Sentences?" 40 JOURNAL OF THE AMERICAN GERIATRICS SOCIETY 722–726 (July 1992); Marshall B. Kapp, "Restrictive State Advance Directive Statutes: Risk Management Implications," 13 JOURNAL OF HEALTHCARE RISK MANAGEMENT 14–18 (Winter 1993).

47. Lawrence Markson & Knight Steel, "Using Advance Directives in the Home-Care Setting," 14 GENERATIONS 25–28 (Supplement 1990).

48. M.P. Daly & J. Sobal, "Advanced Directives Among Patients in a House Call Program," 5 JOURNAL OF THE AMERICAN BOARD OF FAMILY PRACTICE 11–15 (January-February 1992).

49. Emergency Cardiac Care Committee and Subcommittees, American Heart Association, "Guidelines for Cardiopulmonary Resuscitation and Emergency Cardiac Care," 268 JOURNAL OF THE AMERICAN MEDICAL ASSOCIATION 2282–2288 (Part VIII) (October 28, 1992).

50. Diane Havlir, Louise Brown, & G. Kay Rousseau, "Do Not Resuscitate Discussions in a Hospital-Based Home Care Program," 37 JOURNAL OF THE AMERICAN GERIATRICS SOCIETY 52–54 (January 1989).

51. Erich H. Loewy, "Decisions to Leave Home: What Will the Neighbors Say?" 36 JOURNAL OF THE AMERICAN GERIATRICS SOCIETY 1143–1146 (December 1988).

52. Patrick P. Coll & David Anderson, "Letter: Advanced Directives for Homebound Patients," 5 JOURNAL OF THE AMERICAN BOARD OF FAMILY PRACTICE 359–60 (May-June 1992).

53. Greg A. Sachs, Steven H. Miles, & Rebekah A. Levin, "Limiting Resuscitation: Emerging Policy in the Emergency Medical System," 114 ANNALS OF INTERNAL MEDICINE 151–154 (January 15, 1991).

54. *Id.*, at 152–153.

55. *Id.*, at 153.

56. American College of Emergency Physicians, "Guidelines for Do Not Resuscitate Orders in the Prehospital Setting," 17 ANNALS OF EMERGENCY MEDICINE 1106–1108 (October 1988).

57. Bruce E. Haynes & James T. Niemann, "Letting Go: DNR Orders in Prehospital Care," 254 JOURNAL OF THE AMERICAN MEDICAL ASSOCIATION 532–533 (July 26, 1985); Sachs, Miles, & Levin, *supra* note 53, at 152.

58. Colorado Revised Statutes, Title 15, Article 18.6.

59. Jerry A. Menikoff, Greg A. Sachs, & Mark Siegler, "Beyond Advance Directives: Health Care Surrogate Laws," 327 NEW ENGLAND JOURNAL OF MEDICINE 1165–1169 (October 15, 1992).

60. Kapp, *supra* note 46; Kapp, *supra* note 46.

61. Judith Areen, "Advance Directives Under State Law and Judicial Decisions," 19 LAW, MEDICINE & HEALTH CARE 91–100 (Spring-Summer 1991).

62. James Bopp & Daniel Avila, "The Due Process Right to Life in Cruzan and Its Impact on Right to Die Law," 53 UNIVERSITY OF PITTSBURGH LAW REVIEW 193 (1991); James Bopp & Daniel Avila, "Perspectives on Cruzan: The Sirens' Lure of Invented Consent: A Critique of Autonomy-Based Surrogate Decisionmaking for Legally Incapacitated Older Persons," 42 HASTINGS LAW JOURNAL 779–815 (March 1991).

63. Dombi, *supra* note 16, at 81.

64. Bernard Lo, Fenella Rouse, & Lauri Dornbrand, "Family Decision-Making on Trial: Who Decides for Incompetent Patients?" 322 NEW ENGLAND JOURNAL OF MEDICINE 1228–1231 (1990).

65. Loewy, *supra* note 51, at 1144.

66. *State* v. *McAfee*, 385 S.E.2d 651 (Ga. 1989).

67. Feinberg, *supra* note 40, at 113.

68. American College of Emergency Physicians, *supra* note 54.

69. Ann M. Montminy, "Decison-Making Authority for Family Caregivers of the Cognitively Impaired Elderly," 7(4) JOURNAL OF COMMUNITY HEALTH NURSING 215–221 (1990).

70. Ann Young, Catherine H. Pignatello, and Marietta B. Taylor, "Who's the Boss? Ethical Conflicts in Home Care," HEALTH

PROGRESS 59–62 (December 1988); Patricia A. Young & Martha Pelaez, "The In-Service Education Program of the Home Health Assembly of New Jersey," 14 GENERATIONS 37–38 (Supplement 1990).

71. P. Elizabeth Abel, "Ethics Committees in Home Health Agencies," 7 PUBLIC HEALTH NURSING 256–259 (December 1990).

72. *Id.*, at 256–257.

73. Joanne Lynn, "Commentary," in CASEBOOK ON THE TERMINATION OF LIFE-SUSTAINING TREATMENT AND THE CARE OF THE DYING (Cynthia B. Cohen, ed.). Bloomington, IN: Indiana University Press (1988), at 123–125.

74. Loewy, *supra* note 51, at 1144.

75. Collopy, Dubler, & Zuckerman, *supra* note 32, at 3.

Ethnic Americans,[1] Long-Term Health Care Providers, and the Patient Self-Determination Act

6

Vernellia R. Randall, R.N., M.S.N., J.D.

R.S. is tired and frightened. As she waits for her family to complete the admission process to the nursing home, she thinks about how it might have been if she had never left her homeland. True, she had left over 60 years ago. But she was a teenager at the time and she remembered. She remembered the respect that everyone gave the elders. Here in America, there was very little respect.

The young man who was talking to her with a slow speech was young enough to be her great-grandchild. Still, he treated her as if she didn't understand English; which, of course, she did. She understood it perfectly; she just hated to speak it. Despite 60 years, her English was still halting. Often, others became frustrated and

---

[1] I reject the designation of "minorities" because of its connotation of subordination. "Ethnic Americans" is used to refer to African-Americans, Asian-Americans, Native Americans, and Hispanic-Americans.

condescending. Anyway, she knew it was best to keep quiet. This was a new situation and who was to know what is to be learned by listening?

The young man called her by her first name. "R., do you have a living will?" She looked up at him—without response. "Well, here," he said, "is information about a living will and the durable power of health care attorney. Basically, the durable power of health care attorney allows someone you pick to make health care decisions for you when you can't make them for yourself. If you become terminally ill or fall into a persistent vegetated state, the living will allows the doctors to stop treatment, if that is what you have instructed them to do."

This is very confusing, she thought. What decision about life was hers to make? Wasn't that a family decision? How was she to read this document written in English? Just as she thought she might ask a question, the young man hurriedly thrust another paper in her hand. "Please sign this. The law requires us to ask you if you have advance directives and give you information about them. This paper is your acknowledgment that you were asked and that you received the information." Ah—the law she thought, as she signed the paper. Everyone knows that whenever the law is involved one had best hold on to one's purse and one's life. Perhaps it is true what they say—that these places are here to help people like her die quicker. Perhaps her children have placed her here to die. This would not have happened in the old country.

INTRODUCTION

In 1990, Congress passed, and President Bush signed, the Patient Self-Determination Act ("PSDA") (Care & Gill, 1991). PSDA requires certain behaviors of every long-term health care facility that receives Medicaid or Medicare. The PSDA requires these facilities to give every patient written information about patient rights regarding treatment decisions and ask every patient, at admission, if they have a living will or durable power of health care attorney.

Congress enacted the PSDA because of individuals like Nancy Cruzan. For seven years Cruzan lived in a persistent vegetative state. The Missouri Supreme Court held that her parents could not have the life support withdrawn. At trial, Cruzan's parents failed to produce "clear and convincing" evidence of her desires. They failed to convince the court that Cruzan would not want to "continue her present existence, hopeless as it is" (Cruzan, 1990). Subsequently, the U.S. Supreme Court held that states could constitutionally require the "clear and convincing" standard for surrogate decisionmaking.

The existence of a living will or durable power of health care attorney may be such "clear and convincing" evidence. The PSDA creates no new rights; rather, it affirms a person's right to "the possession and control of his person, free from all restraint or interference of others, unless by clear and unquestionable authority of law" (White & Fletcher, 1991, p. 412). In enacting the PSDA, Congress intended to assure that every person has a "meaningful opportunity" to make some provision for decisionmaking about health care before she is incapacitated.

CULTURE AND "MEANINGFUL OPPORTUNITY"

Long-term health care providers provide a meaningful opportunity when this provision takes place within the context of the cultural background and values of the particular patient. Merely asking if a person has a living will or durable power of health care attorney may not constitute a meaningful opportunity to execute one. Furthermore, simply giving a person a handout about such documents will be woefully ineffective in helping ethnic Americans understand the uses, benefits, and weaknesses of such documents.

"Culture" is employed in various manners. It has been defined as an "integrated system of learned patterns of behavior, ideas, and products characteristic of a society" (Perkins, 1991). It is a "body of learned values, beliefs, and behaviors that depict a group of people. Culture provides the basic framework by which individuals interpret their surroundings, the behavior of the people around them, and the events that befall them" (Perkins, 1991, p. 72). Many factors decide a person's culture. These include: race, nationality, native language, education, occupation, religion, socioeconomic characteristics, and area of origin (Harwood, 1981a). These factors affect the individual's values, beliefs, and behaviors; and the values, beliefs, or behavior peculiar to a particular subgroup within a culture define a subculture (Perkins, 1991). For centuries, the United States indulged in the myth that all persons coming to the country blended into one great "melting pot" to become Americans. It is true that Americans have dominant cultural similarities that cross all groups. It is also true that this country has always had a diverse population of races, ethnic groups, subcultures, and religions.

By the end of the century, 39% of the American population will be from foreign-born families. At the same time, 50% will be either African-American, Hispanic-American, Asian-American, or Native Americans (Final Report of White House Commission, 1981). America is a "microworld reflecting [the] cultural diversity of the entire world" (Murillo-Rohde, 1980; Ross, 1981).

The PSDA lacks the flexibility to address the issues and concerns of many Americans. In particular, the PSDA is a representation of one subculture—European-American,[2]

---

[2]I use the term "European American" to denote individuals usually called "white." Historically, ethnic Americans have been designated a hyphenated name: "Black-Americans," "Asian-Americans," "Hispanic-Americans." The presumption seemed to be that you would not recognized these individuals as Americans unless we designated them as such. On the other hand, "white" persons need no designation because they are presumed to be

middle-class, and middle-aged. It is based on promoting individual autonomy instead of family involvement and on the use of written communication in education instead of oral or visual communication. It assumes a basic trust in the health care system instead of distrust.

The more a client differs from the cultural prototype (European-American, middle-class, middle-aged) the more likely it is that the PSDA will be ineffective, and the more likely that the PSDA will not help to assure that the person will have a "meaningful opportunity" to exercise "autonomy" regarding death and dying issues. Consequently, long-term health care providers must look to PSDA's goals. When carrying out the act with ethnic Americans, they must go beyond the bare requirements of the law. If long-term health care providers don't consider cultural differences when they carry out the PSDA, the goals of PSDA will

---

Americans. Consequently, linguistically "white" maintains a position of power.

> White people didn't bother to define themselves racially in any particular way until rather recently. According to usage historian Stuart Berg Flexner, general references to "white men" entered the language only in the 1830s, and didn't gain wide usage until the Civil War. What did whites call themselves until then? They called themselves "people" or "citizens." In other words, they occupied, unchallenged, the center of their racial universe, and needed no further definition of the sort assigned to such outsiders as Indian "savages" or black slaves. "White" became an important term at the time of Emancipation; a reaction to the power threat presented by another racial group." (Freud, 1989, p. a23)

It would be "nice" if no designations at all were needed, but the reality of the situation requires us to discuss the needs of specific ethnic groups. I used the term European, rather than Anglo-Saxon, to provide balance with the other designation; that is, an identification of the geographic region from which the original ancestors migrated.

not be met, and their activities will become nothing more than legal busywork.

IMPLEMENTING THE PSDA WITH ETHNIC AMERICANS

Culture plays a prominent role in the decision and behaviors involved in decision making about death and dying. Culture affects the type of communication that a person prefers and can understand. Culture affects an individual's values and attitudes toward death and dying, toward the body, and religious beliefs. Culture affects how individuals select, perceive, and evaluate health care providers. It influences beliefs about the family's role in life decisions.

Communication

How different cultures communicate is very important. Different linguistic groups see and conceive reality differently (Quesada, 1976). Thus, ethnic Americans' views of death, dying, and advance directives will be shaped by the language they use. Communication and language barriers will exist to the extent that a person's primary language is not based on English.

For example, despite the fact that many Mexican-Americans are bilingual, quite a few speak little or no English. In the Mexican-American culture, like other Hispanic-American cultures, there is significant emphasis placed on paternalistic dependence. The average Mexican-American establishes different *patron-peon* relationships for different activities. However, she nevertheless expects a certain amount of respect (*dignidad*) even when a *patron* is dealing with a *peon*. The Mexican-American patient who is simply given a culturally nonspecific document without explanation may feel that she is being treated as another body— with no *dignidad* (Quesada, 1976).

Language and communication barriers can extend beyond the question of how language shapes reality. There are problems of oral versus written communication. The PSDA only requires a facility to provide patients with written information about advance directives. This emphasis on written communication ignores the fact that many individuals' preferred method of receiving information is through oral or visual communication. If long-term health care facilities don't develop educational programs based on oral and visual communication, these persons will, at best, be inadequately served. Furthermore, simply providing information (written, oral, or visual) does not ensure knowledge or understanding. The law takes a minimalist approach to communication. This approach will be completely inadequate with persons from cultural backgrounds that are not middle-class and European-American.

Expressed language, whether written or oral, is a major source of conflict and misunderstanding in intercultural situations (Ross, 1991). For instance, an inability to understand the expressions of others, or to be understood by others, can be a major source of frustration for ethnic Americans. This becomes a particular problem when a person is admitted to a long-term health care facility. Depression, frustration, and embarrassment may cause even persons with efficiency in English to revert to their native language.

Culture also influences the forms of response in conversation. (Ross, 1991). For example, long-term health care providers should not consider a Hispanic-American's lengthy response to a question inappropriate. The Hispanic-American is merely attempting to put his or her concerns in the framework of the total situation (Ross, 1991). Similarly, when discussing advance directives with Asian-Americans, a long-term health care provider may give more information than they receive. Asian-Americans may refrain from divulging personal information to strangers and will simply answer "yes" or "no" to questions (Gould-Martin & Ngin, 1981; Ross, 1991). Asking a Filipino-American if they understand a question, or if they have an advance directive, may elicit a hesitant "yes" or only silence, since Filipino

Americans try to avoid giving a direct (and consequently painful) "no." While some cultures, such as European-American, view silence as a lack of understanding or knowledge, members of other cultures (i.e., Western Apache Indians) rely on silence in unaccustomed situations. "For a stranger entering an alien society, knowledge of when *not* to speak may be as basic . . . as knowledge of what to say" (Basso, 1970, p. 215). Thus, long-term health care providers should not assume ignorance or lack of understanding merely from the presence of conversational silence.

Similarly, a patient's affect and approach will differ across cultures. For instance, Samoan-Americans and Haitian-Americans may be stoical in their emotional response. Culturally, they consider themselves able to bear life's circumstances without complaint (Ross, 1991). However, Haitian-Americans might become quite emotional in response to any discussion that they interpret as meaning that death is imminent (Laguerre, 1981). Filipino-Americans may find the professional approach of some long-term health care providers to be cold and disconcerting. Filipino-Americans expect warmth and a personal attitude in the delivery of health care (Ross, 1991). Filipino-Americans are also likely to be overt in their emotional responses to grief and distress.

Finally, culture influences the topics that a person considers appropriate for conversation among strangers. European-Americans place a high value on giving patients all the information and allowing them to make the decision (informed consent). The principles of autonomy and informed consent form the theoretical basis for advance directives and the PSDA. However, members of some cultures believe that the family should shield their loved ones from a bad prognosis. Some families may view a discussion of PSDA on admission to a long-term health care facility as conveying news of impending death. A Filipino-American, for example, may find the discussion offensive, and evidence of a failure of the family and the health care provider to shelter him or her from bad news.

Attitudes Toward Death and Dying

Every culture comprehends death and dying differently. For instance, in European-American culture, disclosure of a terminal illness is fundamental to patient care. However, many other cultures reject such disclosure. Mexican-Americans, for example, are very protective of others; many believe that dying persons should be not be told that they are dying. Mexican-Americans could resent the discussion of advance directives if they view it as a discussion of their own impending death (Esberger, 1980; Kalish & Reynolds, 1976). Alaskan Indians, on the other hand, very much want to participate in the planning for their own death (including the time of its occurrence) (Esberger, 1980).

Cultural attitudes toward death influence how individuals will respond to being approached about PSDA. For instance, as compared to European-Americans, Japanese-Americans, and Mexican-Americans, African-Americans expect to and would like to live the longest (Esberger, 1980). In a subculture based on oppression, slavery, poverty, and death, living may be the only hope. Consequently, it's not surprising that African-Americans have a significantly lower suicide rate than European-Americans. African-Americans might resist advance directives as instruments of suicide and may see efforts to encourage their use as efforts to encourage suicide. From 1977 through 1989, by a margin of 20%, European-Americans were consistently more likely than African-Americans to support enactment of "right to die" laws (Wood, 1990). Filipino-Americans may also resist advance directives because they view suicide as shameful. They believe that it brings disrepute on the family.

Japanese-Americans, on the other hand, seem more accepting of death, attaching little importance to the fact that death would end their life's plans. Japanese-Americans are significantly more likely than members of other groups to know someone who committed suicide (Esberger, 1990; Kalish & Reynolds, 1976). Consequently, a discussion of advance directives may not disturb Japanese-Americans as much as other ethnic Americans. Similarly, many Native American groups see death as a part of the normal process of the universe—"an event to be faced with realism and equanimity" (Kunitz & Levy, 1981, p. 384). Chinese-Americans tend to be stoic and fatalistic when faced with terminal illness and death. While impending death is not talked about explicitly, Chinese-Americans may appreciate being given an opportunity to tidy up their affairs. However, a long-term health care provider should conduct such discussion with the permission of the family, or with the patient alone so that the patient can still pretend ignorance with his or her family (Gould-Martin & Ngin, 1981).

Attitudes About the Body

Cultural attitudes about the body affect how a person responds to a provider's actions in implementing the PSDA. Pain and death are physiological phenomena. Ideas of modesty may influence a person's willingness to consider and discuss advance directives with a stranger. For instance, Hispanic-Americans dictate that a person must be modest, even if everyone present is of the same sex (Ross, 1991).

Religious Beliefs

Religious beliefs provide meaning for life and death. Many ethnic Americans believe that suffering, illness, and death are the will of God. For example, Hispanic-Americans view illness, pain, and death as punishments from God for their sinful acts or immoral behaviors while African-Americans' strong religious orientation has helped them survive slavery and oppression (Ross, 1991). These religious beliefs may affect the response a person has to advance directives.

Family's Role in Life Decisions

The PSDA promotes individual autonomy instead of family involvement. Nevertheless, the concept of family may have a particular influence on the carrying out of the PSDA.

The family is the basic societal unit; its members are committed to nurture each other emotionally and physically. Family members are committed to share resources (Smilkstein, 1980). "Family" has different meanings across cultures. To African-Americans, the nuclear family may extend to include grandparents, uncles, aunts, cousins, nieces, nephews, and others. Hispanic-Americans may also refer to the children's godparents as part of the nuclear family. Native Americans may have several "mothers," as the Native American grandmother takes primary responsibility for the care of a child (Ross, 1991). Long-term health care professionals must know cultural differences in kinship terms, in role expectations, and in the role of the family in major decisionmaking.

Different cultural priorities may modify the degree to which families are involved in treatment withdrawal decisions. Some cultures may find a method of personal decisionmaking that focuses on the individual, instead of on the family, particularly offensive. For Mexican-Americans, Native Americans, Haitian-Americans, Puerto Ricans, and Chinese-Americans, illness is a family affair (Gould-Martin & Ngin, 1981; Harwood, 1981b; Kunitz & Levy, 1991; Laguerre, 1981; Ross, 1991; Schreiber & Homiak, 1981). Family members are involved in the patient's medical decisions and care (Gould-Martin, 1981).

Ultimately, approaching an individual or family with the PSDA upon admission to a long-term health care facility may affect how the family and individual respond to placement in the facility. Being admitted to a long-term health care facility is stressful for any person. It is particularly stressful for individuals who come from ethnic groups that strongly prefer home care to institutional care (Harwood, 1981a; Ross, 1991).

Chinese-Americans, Haitian-Americans, Mexican-Americans, and rural African-Americans prefer home care, while urban African-Americans and Navajo Native Americans do not hold such a preference[3] (Harwood, 1981a). Among those groups who prefer home care, their apprehension is that their family members will die alone in a long-term health care facility. For instance, many Native American groups believe that the spirit of their loved one cannot leave the body until the family is there (Ross, 1991). A discussion of advance directives at the time of admission may affirm their apprehension that they are leaving their family member to face dying alone.

Trust of the Health Care System

The PSDA presupposes a trust in the health care system. It presupposes that a patient will interpret the discussion of advance directives as an educational activity or, at the very worst, a neutral activity. However, many individuals in our society distrust the health care system. Studies have suggested that the more contact individuals in a country have with health care providers, the more negative their attitudes will be toward health care providers and services (Champion, Austin, & Tzeng, 1990). Consequently, after years of neglect and culturally insensitive care there is often a deep distrust of the health care system. This is true even when those providing the health care are of the same ethnic community (*Forgotten Americans*, 1990). African-Americans' distrust is rooted in slavery, sharecropping, peonage, lynchings, Jim Crow laws, disenfranchisement, residential segregation, job discrimination, insufficient health care, and inappropriate scientific experimentation (Cary, 1992; Jones, 1992), African-Americans may feel that long-term health care providers will use the advance directives to terminate care for them sooner than they would for European Americans. They may view a discussion of advance

---

[3]The high percentage of urban African-American women in the work force probably accounts for this population's lack of preference for home care. The Navajo's fear of spirit contamination from the dead accounts for their lack of preference.

directives at the time of admission as an affirmation of their views.

Many Southeast Asian-Americans identify the health care system with death (Uba, 1992). Many Hispanic-Americans distrust the community health care system. They do not take advantage of the limited services available, apparently because of their perception that agencies exploit low-income people. They also perceive providers as obstacles to receiving any meaningful help (Mettger & Freimuth, 1990).

Historically, Hispanic-Americans, and particularly Mexican-Americans, have not had access to good housing, schooling, or health services. Neglect combined with bigotry and discrimination has encouraged Hispanic-Americans to be suspicious of the health care system (Schreiber & Homiak, 1981). Unquestionably, a person's advance directive may be vague and subject to interpretation. The distrust that some ethnic Americans feel for the health care system may be reaffirmed when health care providers, families, and courts debate over the meaning of an advance directive.

SUMMARY

Long-term health care providers frequently interact with persons who subscribe to beliefs and practices that are very different from their own. They will not be effective in meeting the goals of the PSDA if they do not bridge the gap. They can do this by becoming aware of the differences; by being ready to identify them by exploring them; and by changing their behaviors to reflect this understanding. Long-term health care providers who work with ethnic Americans have the opportunity to turn the experience of difference and discomfort into a learning situation both for themselves and the patient.

The law was designed with certain assumptions in mind: that individual autonomy and individual decisionmaking has the highest priority; that written communications about PSDA will provide a person with meaningful opportunity to enact a living will or durable power of attorney; and that admissions to a hospital or a long-term health care facility are the best opportunities for such education.

What the Congress ought to have done was to build alternate requirements into the PSDA. Long-term health care providers will need to do more than the Congress required; they will need to develop ways to give each client a culturally meaningful opportunity to direct treatment decisions. Long-term health care providers should use community resources and tools to enhance their understanding of ethnic Americans.

SUGGESTIONS

Ask the Patient

The long-term health care provider should seek the patient's opinion about what is culturally appropriate whenever possible. This is important because cultural patterns are not predictive of individual behavior. Ethnic variations in practices, beliefs, and reactions are complicated by differences in rural versus urban background, differences in sex, and differences in educational experience.

Explain in Detail

The long-term health care provider should understand that persons from many cultures want a full explanation. This is true even though they may have difficulty in understanding the explanation. The long-term health care provider should avoid using technical language. The provider should avoid rushing the discussion.

Use Culturally Specific Communication

If written communication is used, handouts should be provided in the patient's language. The handout should be more than a translation of the English document. It should be culturally specific and tailored to the concerns of the ethnic population.

Provide Opportunities for Discussion

Long-term health care providers should give ethnic American patients and families the opportunity to discuss fully advance directives and living wills (Fletcher & White, 1991).

Provide a Translator if Necessary

If the patient and the family members prefer to speak in a language other than English, the long-term health care facility should accommodate them. This can be done either by speaking the preferred language or by using an accurate and sympathetic translator. A translator should never be a stranger from the waiting room; neither should the person be the patient's minor child.

Determine the Language of Choice

Even for those who are nominally bilingual, the inability of the health care providers to converse in their dominant language may be viewed as a form of ethnocentrism (Schreiber & Homiak, 1981). However, the provider should not assume that an ethnic American necessarily wants to carry on the conversation in a language other than English. If the language ability is not immediately apparent, the long-term health care provider should ask what language the patient prefers to use. Furthermore, the provider should not assume that ethnic Americans speak the official language of the country of origin. For instance, when asked if they speak French, most Haitians will answer "yes." However, only the elites in Haiti speak French; most Haitian-Americans speak Haitian Creole (Laguerre, 1981).

Be Patient

Long-term health care providers must allow English speaking ethnic Americans enough time to find the proper English words. Furthermore, the provider must not show exasperation over the ethnic American's manner of speaking English (Laguerre, 1981).

Be Respectful of the Family

The long-term health care provider should express his or her respect and caring for the family members. For instance, a quiet and unhurried but purposeful demeanor is reassuring to Southeast Asian-Americans because it characterizes "wisdom, good judgment and dignity" (Muecke, p. 433, 1983, p. 433).

Be Respectful of Personal Space

The long-term health care provider should understand the patient's cultural feelings about being touched. That is, if the patient comes from a culture that demands personal space, then the long-term health care provider should respect that space by minimizing touching.

Use Direct Eye Contact

When speaking with the patient and family members, the long-term health care provider should position his or herself at their eye level. The exchange should be informative and not rushed.

Encourage Participation

The long-term health care provider should welcome those relatives, friends, and other advisers whom the patient wants to participate in the discussion and the decisionmaking.

Respect the Elderly

Ethnic Americans who originate from kin-based or peasant societies generally accord greater respect to the elderly than do members of the European American subculture. A long-term health care provider who is younger than the patient should adopt toward most elderly ethnic Americans an attitude of greater respect and seriousness than they might typically display. A long-term health care provider who is older than the patient will need to encourage younger ethnic Americans to reduce the reticence the patient might feel because of the relationship.

Don't be Overly Familiar

Don't use first names with patients. Many ethnic Americans interpret this as a lack of respect. African-Americans, in particular, interpret the use of first names as a continuation of the master-servant relationship (Jackson, 1981).

To adjust to the diversity in the United States and to actualize the goals of the PSDA, long-term health care providers must adopt a cross-cultural viewpoint. They must:

- Appreciate ethnic Americans both as individuals and as members of culturally distinct groups;
- Identify the cultural beliefs and practices of ethnic Americans that differ from their own;
- Understand how culture has affected their own biases; and,
- Modify the carrying out of the PSDA to incorporate differing beliefs and practices (Ross, 1981).

REFERENCES

Basso, K. (1970). To give up on words: Silence in Western Apache culture. *Southwestern Journal of Anthropology, 26,* 215, 213–230.

Care, F. H., & Gill, B. A. (1991). *The Patient Self-Determination Act: Implementation issues and opportunities: A white paper of the Annenberg Washington Program.* Washington, DC: Annenberg Washington Program.

Cary, L. (1992, April 6). Why it's not just paranoia: An American history of "plans" for blacks. *Newsweek,* p. 23.

Champion, V. L., Austin, J. K., & Tzeng, O.C.S. (1990). Relationship between Cross-cultural Health Attitudes and Community Health Indicators, *Public Health Nursing, 7,* 243–250, 249.

Cruzan, V. Director, Missouri Department of Health, 110 S. Ct. 2841, (1990).

Esberger, K. K. (1980). Dying and the aged, *Journal of Gerontological Nursing, 11*, 11–15.

Final Report of Select White House Commission on Immigration and Refuge Policy, Second Semi-Annual Report to Congress, Washington, D.C. US Government Printing Office (1981), Serial No. J. 97-38.

Fletcher, J. C., & White, M. L. (1991). Patient Self-Determination Act to Become Law: How Should Institutions Prepare? *Bio Law: A Legal and Ethical Reporter on Medicine, Health Care and Bioengineering, 2.*

Freud, C. P. (1989, February 7). Rhetorical questions: The power of, and behind, a name. *The Washington Post*, p. a23.

Forgotten Americans: Special report on medical care for blacks (1990). *American Health*, 52–56.

Gould-Martin, K., & Ngin, C. (1981). Chinese Americans. In A. Harwood (Ed.), *Ethnicity and medical care* (pp. 130–144). Cambridge: Harvard University Press.

Harwood, A. (1981a) Guidelines for culturally appropriate health care. In A. Harwood (Ed.), *Ethnicity and Medical Care* (pp. 452–507). Cambridge: Harvard University Press.

Harwood, A. (1981b). Mainland Puerto Rican. In A. Harwood (Ed.), *Ethnicity and medical care* (pp. 397–473). Cambridge: Harvard University Press.

Jackson, J. J. (1981). Urban Black Americans. In A. Harwood (Ed.), *Ethnicity and medical care* (pp. 37–130). Cambridge: Harvard University Press.

Jones, J. (1992). The Tuskegee legacy: AIDS and the black community (twenty years after: The legacy of the Tuskegee Syphilis Study). *Hastings Center Report, 22*, 38–40.

Kunitz, S. J., & Levy, J. E. (1981). Navajos. In A. Harwood (Ed.), *Ethnicity and medical care* (pp. 337–388). Cambridge: Harvard University Press.

Laguerre, M. S. (1981). Haitian Americans. In A. Harwood (Ed.), *Ethnicity and medical care* (pp. 191–206). Cambridge: Harvard University Press.

Mettger, W., & Freimuth, V. S. (1990). Is there a hard-to-reach audience? *Public Health Reports, 105*, 232–238.

Muecke, M. A. (1983). Caring for Southeast Asian refugee patients in the USA. *American Journal of Public Health, 73*, 431, 433.

Murillo-Rohde, I. (1980). *Unique needs of ethnic minority clients in a multiracial society: A socio-cultural perspective in affirmative action: Toward quality nursing care for a multiracial society*. (ANA Pub. No. M-24 2500).

Perkins, H. S. (1991). Cultural differences and ethical issues in the problem of autopsy requests. *Texas Medicine/The Journal*, *87*, 72–77.

Quesada, G. M. (1976). Language and communication barriers for health delivery to minority groups. *Social Science and Medicine*, *10*, 323, 324.

Ross, M. R. (1991). Societal/cultural views regarding death and dying. *Topics in Clinical Nursing*, *5*, 1–16.

Schreiber, J. M., & Homiak, J. P. (1981). Mexican Americans. In A. Harwood (Ed.), *Ethnicity and medical care* (pp. 264–329). Cambridge: Harvard University Press.

Smilkstein, G. (1980). The cycle of family function: A conceptual model for family medicine. *The Journal of Family Practice*, 223, 224.

Uba, L. (1992). Cultural barriers to health care for southeast Asian refugees. *Public Health Reports*, *107*, 544, 546.

White, M. L., & Fletcher, J. C. (1991). The Patient Self-Determination Act: On balance, more help than hindrance. *Journal of the American Medical Association*, *266*, 410.

Wood, F. (Ed.). (1990). *An American profile: Attitude and Behavior of the American People, 1972–1989* (pp. 627–628). Detroit: Gale Research.

Liability Issues and Assessment of Decisionmaking Capability in Nursing Home Patients

7

Marshall B. Kapp, J.D., M.P.H.

In health care delivery generally, a free-floating fear of legal liability dominates the thinking of many health care providers. This tends to motivate them toward attitudes and behavior that, in the providers' perception, at least, minimizes risks of harm to the patient and associated risks of legal and financial loss to the providers. That is, apprehension about liability makes providers risk-averse. This phenomenon often results in high costs in terms of patient autonomy, patient well-being, and wasted patient and societal economic resources.[1]

In nursing homes especially, this risk aversion contributes, in this author's opinion, to a bias toward reliance (and frequently overreliance) on surrogates—particularly family members with or without explicit legal authority—to make decisions. Often this practice substitutes for a careful assessment of the patient's own functional capacity to engage in a rational decisionmaking process, at least in certain issues. Physicians and nursing home administrators generally have a much greater anxiety about a patient's relatives as potential malpractice plaintiffs than they do about the patient herself taking on that role. Thus, deference to family involvement in many cases trumps patient involvement where there is any question raised about the patient's decisionmaking capacity.

Health care providers sometimes cite liability fears as a pretext for rationalizing conduct that actually is driven more by professional bias (e.g., old, frail nursing home patients must be unable to make decisions, or else they would be young, healthy, and attending professional conferences) or administrative convenience. This rationalization may be conscious or subconscious. It undeniably is much more efficient to deal with an articulate relative than to do a thorough evaluation on an impaired older nursing home patient; to tailor specific decisionmaking processes to the patient's specific capabilities in order to assist the patient to maximize limited but real capabilities; and to document all of these efforts. Nonetheless, this is not a categoric description of provider behavior. In many instances, liability fears are sincerely felt by physicians and nursing home administrators who believe that their options for delivering quality care that respects the patient's autonomy and dignity are unduly constrained.

This article briefly outlines: 1) physician and nursing home administrator perceptions concerning their liability risks regarding assessment of decisionmaking capacity and resulting behavioral consequences; 2) a perspective on those liability risks; 3) strategies for managing those risks that are consistent with patient autonomy and welfare; and 4) public policy options for rectifying current deficiencies in assessing capacity in the nursing home environment, where deficiencies are attributable to anxiety about legal liability.

It should be noted that much of this discussion applies with full force to frail, dependent elders residing in the community. Since nursing homes are unique, total institutions housing more than 1.5 million Americans, however, they receive special attention in this article.

PERCEPTIONS AND BEHAVIORAL CONSEQUENCES

Most health care providers, especially physicians, pay relatively little attention to the issue of decisionmaking capacity or its liability implications except in cases of invasive, risky, or experimental interventions. Thus, there generally is likely to be less concern about this issue in nursing home settings. Most decisions here center more around mundane, nondramatic matters, such as what time to eat or what clothes to wear, than in the acute care hospital medically oriented environment.[2]

Also, most nursing home administrators are far more anxious about regulatory pressures (e.g., the threat of delicensure or decertification from the Medicaid or Medicare programs) than about the relatively remote (to this point, at least) risk of tort litigation. There is scant regulatory guidance for nursing home administrators or the physicians who care for patients within their facilities on the assessment of decisional capacity issue. Federal and state laws essentially defer without comment to state guardianship law,[3] which in most jurisdictions is itself quite murky.[4]

Even when the decision that needs to be made is one that the physician and nursing home administrator take seriously (i.e., that entails some degree of intrusion or risk), little careful thought is devoted to assessing the nonobjecting patient's capacity.[5,6] This is particularly true if surrogate decisionmakers are available and everyone is in agreement on the desired course of action. Since the physician's and administrator's legal anxiety focuses on the family as potential plaintiff, a cooperative family puts the providers' anxiety at ease and quenches the thirst for further reflection on the patient's capacity. This complacency may be strengthened by the physician's and administrator's reliance on the "responsible party" status of a relative. A "responsible party" is one who voluntarily agrees to assure payment for a patient's care, and the 1987 Omnibus Budget Reconciliation Act (OBRA 1987) now forbids facilities from requiring new patients to have a "responsible party."[7] Nevertheless, many physicians and nursing home administrators are under the mistaken impression that the "responsible party" also automatically acquires medical and other decisionmaking authority on the patient's behalf.[8]

Sometimes there is a question about patient decisional capacity and no surrogate is reasonably available, or there is disagreement (among rival surrogates, between surrogate and patient, or between surrogate and provider) that is not resolved through an informal communication and negotiation process. In such circumstances, many physicians and nursing home administrators are fearful of liability for proceeding on the sole basis of the patient's own express wishes (assuming the patient can even express wishes). In these scenarios, the physician or administrator may insist—in the name of risk management—on judicial appointment of a formal substitute decisionmaker (i.e., a guardian or conservator). This approach is contrary to the "least restrictive alternative" position, stating that most cases involving decisionmaking for persons of questionable functional status are better dealt with outside of the court system.[9,10]

Nevertheless, in situations in which the informal process of communication and negotiation will not work, the judicial forum may indeed be a less restrictive alternative than abandoning the questionably competent patient's well-being to an absence of advocacy and oversight. It is not the ultimate resort to the courts that is per se objectionable, but rather a practice of automatic reliance on the pacifying protection of a judicial decree, instead of first exploring available nonjudicial options for safeguarding both the patient and provider.

Especially in nursing homes, where the available pool of potential guardians/conservators often is quite shallow, an undue preoccupation with liability may result in defaulting a decision to crisis mode. The patient may be transformed to a hospital where medical intervention occurs on the basis of the emergency exception to the ordinary informed

consent rule. The ability to shift the most difficult decisional capacity cases to other providers—hospitals, hospices, and, in extreme cases, mental institutions—is a fundamental characteristic of nursing home care.

Admittedly, the aforementioned description of physician
and nursing home administrator behavior rests heavily on
the author's impressions. The phenomenon of defensive
medicine in the context of assessing decisional capacity
among nursing home patients has not been systematically
studied and empirically verified; careful investigation of
this behavior needs to be conducted.

It should also be acknowledged that physician behavior
in assessing the capacity of nursing home residents (as well
as community dwellers) is influenced by the traditional fru-
gality of third-party payers in compensating physicians for
rendering cognitive services. This economic disincentive re-
inforces the negative impact of legal apprehension. The effects, if any, of implementation of Resource-Based Relative
Value Scales for physician payment on physician conduct
in this realm should be evaluated.

LIABILITY RISKS IN PERSPECTIVE

It is perceptions of the law that most strongly influence
provider behavior. Those perceptions need to be compared
to the realistic legal risks so that efforts can be made to reconcile the former with the latter as much as possible. In
this light, it must be kept in mind that malpractice litigation brought against nursing homes or their physicians in
the United States thus far has constituted a negligible frac-
tion of the claims brought against physicians or institutions in acute and ambulatory care settings.[11] Further, virtually none of the cases that have been filed against nursing
homes or their physicians have been based on shortcom-
ings in assessing a patient's decisional capacity. There are
at least two explanations for this phenomenon.

First, there are barriers in the operation of the legal system itself to the successful prosecution of such claims. A successful negligence claim requires, among other things, proof by a preponderance of evidence that the plaintiff suffered a compensable injury. It must be established conclusively that the injury was proximately or directly caused by the defendant's violation of duty. It would be difficult, if not impossible, for most nursing home patients to satisfy the burden of proof that a physician's professionally substandard assessment of decisional capacity proximately caused the patient substantial injuries of the sort that the tort system is intended to compensate. These injuries include future lost earnings, extra medical bills, and foregone economic opportunities.

In the same vein, we live in what Elias Cohen[12] has called a claims-based society. Even if a person's legal rights have been violated, ordinarily no redress is forthcoming unless the wronged individual personally activates the legal apparatus to demand the remedy. Most nursing home patients may lack the physical and mental ability and energy to successfully seek out redress for injuries suffered through inattention to or impropriety in the assessment of decisional capacity.

Where the family or others have acted as decisionmakers on behalf of the patient, they are legally estopped from later claiming that they lacked legal authority to fulfill the substitute decisionmaker's role. Thus, one cannot make decisions on the patient's behalf and then decide retrospectively to hold the provider liable for violating the patient's autonomy.

Further, even if a claim were properly brought procedurally and the evidentiary hurdles of damage and causation were somehow overcome, courts are extremely reluctant to second-guess the judgment of a health care provider—especially a physician—concerning a patient's decisionmaking capacity. Courts presume that the physician has a special expertise and experience in conducting such assessments. Most courts also presume that any particular assessment is based on careful first-hand observation of the patient at the time the professional judgment about capacity is rendered, a database that the judge knows he or she cannot replicate after the fact. (The accuracy of these presumptions, of course, is debatable.) Judicial deference to physician expertise is likely to be strongest in the nursing home arena. There is a presumption that the nursing home physician has a long and rich history of clinical observations upon which to predicate the assessment of a particular patient's decisional capacity.

RISK MANAGEMENT STRATEGIES

Even the very small legal risks associated with decisional capacity assessments in nursing homes can be strategically managed and contained. The most important risk management activities in this area include development and implementation of written institutional protocols for capacity assessment; more careful, thorough assessments utilizing clear criteria and focused on functional ability to make specific kinds of decisions; conscientious data gathering as part of the decisional capacity assessment process, including the observations of family members and all participants in the patient's care team: liberal use of professional consultants for the most challenging cases; and complete, timely documentation of decisional capacity assessments, including the underlying data and the physician's reasoning process. In addition, the physician conducting the assessment may believe that the patient is capable of making the decision in question, but feels legally intimidated to indulge the preferences of the protesting family instead. In such cases, the physician and nursing home administrator ordinarily should shift to the family the burden of overcoming the legal presumption of the patient's decisionmaking capacity. They should inform the family that, in the absence of a court order appointing someone as the patient's guardian, the physician and administrator will follow the patient's wishes. So informed in advance and given an opportunity to initiate judicial intervention, the family cannot be heard later to complain that the physician or administrator acted improperly in relying on the patient's decision.

Long-term care providers, particularly physicians, must become better informed about, and more comfortable in working with, advance directives like durable powers of attorney that purport to delegate decisionmaking authority in a manner consistent with the patient's wishes.[13] Durable powers of attorney for health care are legal documents expressly authorized by statute in almost all of the states, allowing a capable patient to delegate to an agent the authority to make medical decisions on the patient's behalf. This device offers the patient the advantage of extending her autonomy, and the physician or nursing home administrator the advantage of a capable human being with whom informative discussions may be held about the patient's care and who possesses legal authority to make decisions.

Most durable powers of attorney are springing in nature, i.e., they are intended to become effective only upon the decisionmaking incapacity of the principal who delegated the authority. Hence, their use does not obviate the need for the physician to make a determination about the patient's decisionmaking capacity. Use of such directives, though, should reduce the liability exposure of the physician and administrator for determining when conditions have been met, in terms of the principal's incapacity, for the power to spring to the designated agent. Some older persons are comfortable delegating decisionmaking authority to others (usually children) without putting such delegation into words.[14] The physician and nursing home administrator should respect and rely on such delegation without fear of legal repercussions, assuming that the voluntary, informed nature of the delegation has been ascertained and recorded.

PUBLIC POLICY OPTIONS

Several policy options are arguable for correcting any skewing of the decisionmaking capacity assessment process that now results from undue apprehension of legal liability in the long-term care context. First, the federal and/or state governments could promulgate and enforce command and control regulations that very strictly prescribe assessment criteria and procedures and that provide immunity against lawsuits for following the governmental protocols in good faith. This strategy offers the virtues of clarity, definitude, and uniformity, as well as the assurance that the capacity issue will be taken seriously. However, these advantages would be gained at the price of much professional discretion, judgment, and opportunity for flexibility.

Second, instead of governmental fiat, it likely would be more effective for public and private third-party payers to provide financial incentives for physicians and nursing home administrators to take more seriously the decisionmaking capacity issue. For example, payers might condition payment for specific services on the presence of documentation that the service in question was consented to by someone (the patient or a surrogate) who had the mental capacity and legal competency to render such consent.[15] Such direct economic incentives are likely to trump freefloating anxiety about liability risks in shaping provider behavior.

In this vein, Congress in 1990 enacted the "Patient Self-Determination Act" introduced by Senators Danforth and Moynihan and Representative Levin. This bill created an economic incentive (i.e., continued Medicaid funding) for states to require, by statute, that health care institutions have written policies and procedures in place addressed to the process of making difficult medical decisions. States have to ensure that providers educate patients about their rights and options. Presumably, one upshot of the bill will be greater attention to assessment of decisional capacity in nursing homes.

Third, the government could create a private civil right of action (perhaps brought by the long-term care ombudsman on the patient's behalf and/or a regulatory sanction (e.g., civil fine) against the nursing home for too readily deferring to a surrogate decisionmaker without adequate assessment of the patient's own capacity. Physicians and administrators routinely slight the autonomy rights of nursing home patients because of the fear of legal risks threatening them at the hands of the patients' families. Those fears, and the undesirable behavior they inspire, could be counterbalanced by legal risks weighing in the other direction. This strategy would not, of course, alleviate the legal anxiety that engenders many of the problems cited in the first place. It might, however, channel some of that anxiety into more desirable behavior.

CONCLUSIONS

There are many residents of nursing homes who lack the functional capacity to make and express autonomous decisions about serious life issues. These vulnerable individuals need the protection provided by well-intentioned substitute decisionmakers.

A large number of individuals receiving long term care, however, are capable—especially with appropriate assistance—of making and expressing many important choices in a meaningful, autonomous manner. We must develop better professional methodologies for distinguishing between the former and latter groups. These methodologies should be driven by clinical criteria and ethical values about the reach and limits of personal autonomy and society's duty to protect those at risk. Disproportionate and misplaced apprehension of legal liability has no rightful place in the decisional capacity assessment process.

ACKNOWLEDGMENTS

An earlier version of this paper was presented at a Working Conference on Assessment of Decision-Making Capability in Long-Term Care, held at the University of Minnesota, December 17–18, 1989.

REFERENCES

1. Kapp, M. Ethics vs. fear of malpractice. Generations 1985: 10 (Winter): 18–20.

2. Kane, R.A., Caplan, A. Eds. Everyday ethics: resolving dilemmas in nursing home life. New York: Springer Publishing Company, 1990.

3. Title 42 Code of Federal Regulations Section 483.10 (a) (3)

4. American Bar Association Commission on Legal Problems of the Elderly and Commission on the Mentally Disabled. Guardianship: an agenda for reform. Washington, DC: American Bar Association. 1989.

5. Sprung, C. Informed consent in theory and practice: legal and medical perspectives on the informed consent doctrine and a proposed reconceptualization. Critical Care Medicine 1989; 17: 1346.

6. Gurian, B., Baker, E., Jacobson S., Lagertborn, B., Watts P. Informed consent for neuroleptics with elderly patients in two settings. Journal of the American Geriatrics Society 1990: 38:37.

7. Title 42 United States Code Sections 1395e-3 (c) (5) (A) (ii), 1396r (c) (5) (A) (ii)

8. Kapp, M. Responsible parties, power of attorney relationships. Provider 1989: 15:25.

9. Kloezen, S., Fitten, I., Steinberg, A. Assessment of treatment decision-making capacity in a medically ill patient. Journal of the American Geriatrics Society 1988: 36: 1055.

10. Annas, G., Densberger, J. Competence to refuse medical treatment: autonomy vs. paternalism. University of Toledo Law Review 1984: 15: 561.

11. Kapp, M.B. Preventing malpractice in long-term care: strategies for risk management. New York: Springer Publishing Company, 1987.

12. Cohen, E. Nursing homes and the least-restrictive environment doctrine. In: Kapp M.B., Pies, H., Doudera, A.E. Eds. Legal and ethical aspects of health care for the elderly. Ann Arbor: Health Administration Press. 1985.

13. Swidler, R. The health care agent: protecting the choices and interests of patients who lack capacity. NY Law School Journal of Human Rights 1988: 6: 1.

14. Kapp, M.B. Medical empowerment of the elderly. Hastings Center Report 1989: 9: 5.

15. Kapp, M. Enforcing patient preferences: linking payment for medical care to informed consent. JAMA 1989: 261: 1935.

State Statutes Limiting Advance Directives: Death Warrants or Life Sentences?

8

Marshall B. Kapp, J.D., M.P.H.

This is a propitious time for a careful examination and evaluation of state statutes throughout the United States that deal with the subject of decisionmaking about life-sustaining medical treatments (LSMT) and with the execution of advance directives regarding such decisions. Within constitutional boundaries that it enunciated or implied concerning individual liberty rights, the Supreme Court in the 1990 *Cruzan* case[1] gave the various states broad leeway to set their own procedural requirements in this arena, at least insofar as surrogate decisionmaking on behalf of decisionally incapacitated patients was involved. Largely in response to *Cruzan* (although the initiative predates this judicial decision),[2] Congress enacted the Patient Self-Determination Act (PSDA) as part of the Omnibus Budget Reconciliation Act (OBRA) of 1990.[3] This Act requires, among other things,[4] that each state develop and distribute a written document spelling out its own public policies on LSMT decisionmaking, within the confines of which individual health care institutions must develop and distribute their own policies.

During the past two decades, a strong legal and ethical consensus has developed in favor of shared medical decisionmaking premised on a process of communication and negotiation over time among the mentally capable patient, family members and significant friends, physician, and other members of the health care team. Such a process best embodies the important value of individual patient autonomy. Serious problems arise, though, when the patient is unable, either physically or mentally, to participate meaningfully in the discussion. This is particularly true where the patient has not previously provided, by explicit words or a pattern of conduct from which reasonable inferences may be drawn, a clear indication of personal preferences concerning LSMT under various conditions. In an attempt to mitigate some of the ethical, psychological, and legal burdens of medical choice falling on the patient's family, friends, and professional caregivers in such difficult circumstances, much emphasis has been placed on encouraging and facilitating timely advance health care planning, including the writing of specific advance directives, while individuals still retain their decisionmaking capacity.

Many state legislatures prior to 1990 had already enacted legislation setting out mechanisms for individuals to write and sign advance medical directives, in an attempt to foresee and prepare for a future in which medical decisions may need to be made but in which the patient may no longer be able to make and express autonomous choices personally. Instruction directives (living wills) are documents in which the principal indicates personal preferences and desires concerning the provision or abatement of specific types of medical interventions in the future. Proxy directives (durable powers of attorney), which may be executed separately or in tandem with instruction directives, are used by a principal to name a health care decisionmaking agent with legal authority to act in the future in the contingency that the principal becomes incapacitated. In

light of *Cruzan* and the PSDA, many states in the past several years have reviewed and revised their advance directives legislation; some states have just passed living will,
durable power of attorney, and family consent statutes for
the first time.[5]

A number of forces have combined to encourage enactment of advance directive and family consent legislation.
Statutes in this arena are attractive to physicians and other
health care providers because they supply, or at least are
perceived to supply, a degree of legal immunity where
strict compliance with the letter of statutory requirements
has taken place. The general public overwhelmingly favors
such legislation (although many people fail to take advantage of it) because of a belief, largely fostered by legislators,
that such statutes will enhance patient and family control
over the patient's medical treatment destiny, and reduce
the family's emotional turmoil in crisis circumstances.

In many situations, these desired goals indeed are pro-
moted by enacting statutes at the state level, and effective
legislation in this vein should be supported. However, these
promised objectives often are not realized in fact, and inart-
fully drawn statutes may exacerbate, rather than mitigate,
problems for involved participants.

PROBLEMS WITH SOME STATE STATUTES

Ohio's new statute on LSMT[6] represents (albeit in extreme form) a typical phenomenon: state advance directive
and family consent legislation that, in the guise of promoting autonomous decisionmaking and reducing judicial involvement in private matters, is likely to have precisely the
opposite effect in practice. In her comprehensive analysis
of state statutes in this sphere, a respected scholar has
concluded:

> Most of these statutes include fairly rigorous standards for
> preparing a binding directive. Many statutes provide, for ex-
> ample, that a directive becomes binding only if and when

the patient is determined to be terminally ill—and typically that determination must be by more than one physician. In some states a directive is legally binding only if, after the on-set of terminal illness but before the onset of incompetence (a fleeting moment for some patients), the patient reaffirms the directive. Increasingly, physicians and lawyers alike have criticized these statutory models both for their procedural obstacles and for failing to make clear which forms of care are to be foregone and in what circumstances.[7]

Comparing state statutes, Dean Areen observes substan-tial variation in terms of which patients are covered, which treatments may be withdrawn or withheld, which family members are eligible to act as surrogate decisionmakers, and what restraints are placed on the family's ability to make decisions on behalf of the incapacitated patient.[8] The Executive Director of Choice in Dying, the leading national advocacy organization in this sphere, has suggested that ex-isting law on refusal of treatment, advance directives, and decisionmaking by surrogates is "an extraordinary and confusing patchwork . . . The law also . . . ranges from def-erence to private decisions . . . to a considerable amount of state or third-party involvement. . . . The confusion caused by the differences between states is compounded, on occa-sion, by inconsistency even within one state"[9] (p. 92).

For instance, the Ohio statute (as is true of a number of other states) provides legal immunity to a physician who honors a patient's choice to refuse certain LSMT, expressed either through a living will or a surrogate to whom author-ity is delegated under a durable power of attorney, only if there is certification (in many jurisdictions requiring more than one medical opinion) that the patient is terminally ill or in a persistent vegetative state (PVS). Ohio physicians de-siring statutory immunity are mandated to notify specified relatives of their intent to follow the instructions of a living will or authorized agent, and those relatives are invited to file a court challenge within 48 hours. Where a patient is decisionally incapacitated but has not executed an advance directive, many states have family consent statutes that expressively permit specified relatives to make LSMT decisions, but often with severe restrictions imposed. Under the Ohio law, for instance, relatives may consent to the withholding or withdrawal of LSMT for an incapacitated patient who lacks an advance directive only if the patient is terminally ill or has been in a PVS for at least 1 year, and even then a court order is mandated. The Ohio statute, as well as many other state advance directive and family consent provisions, places substantial extra restrictions on the removal of artificial feeding tubes.

State advance directive and family consent statutes that erect complicated, elaborate procedural barriers to the withholding or withdrawal of LSMT, under the pretense of protecting vulnerable patients from victimization at the hands of unscrupulous family members and physicians, are objectionable on several grounds. Instead of authorizing patient and family-desired death warrants delivering persons from unacceptable pain and absence of quality of life, these statutes may operate, in effect, as life sentences imprisoning innocent participants, over their objections, in a medical nightmare.

Damage to Autonomy

First, restrictive state advance directive and family consent statutes, as applied in practice by physicians and other health care providers, impinge on, rather than promote, the decisional autonomy of patient, family, and physician by limiting the situations in which the preferences and values of the patient and family will be honored. For instance, under the Ohio statute and numerous others, a physician does not receive legal immunity for obeying the patient's autonomous, authentic choice—expressed through a living will or durable power of attorney—not to be subjected to continuing LSMT in the event of severe and irreversible dementia falling short of terminal illness or PVS. This absence of express legal immunity would apply even where there is no doubt about the patient's intent, no hint of a conflict of interest, and the physician's ethical and clinical judgment is in accord with the patient and/or family's desire to forego LSMT.

Confusion, Uncertainty, and Unpredictability

Besides damaging the ethical principle of autonomy or self-determination, in most cases without any real corresponding benefit in beneficence or protection from harm, restrictive state advance directive and family consent statutes have other negative effects. They foster terrible confusion, uncertainty, and unpredictability for health care providers and the public concerning their respective rights, obligations, and liabilities. In the last few years, physicians, patients, and families began to become comfortable with an informal process of communication and negotiation among the parties. When the patient no longer retains decisional capacity this process has been guided by the principles of substituted judgment (acting on what the patient would wish, to the extent that the patient's wishes are known or can be inferred) or the best interests of the patient as judged by the other parties. This informal process has led to decisions regarding the limitation of LSMT that, except in very extreme circumstances such as deep and intractable family disagreement, were being implemented without the turmoil and expense of judicial involvement.

Most thoughtful analyses [9,10,11] of the Supreme Court justices' different *Cruzan* opinions argue persuasively that, taken together, these opinions stand for the propositions that:

1) the Fourteenth Amendment due process liberty interest includes the right of a decisionally capable person to make LSMT decisions, presently or prospectively, through an instruction or proxy advance directive, and that a state statute is not necessary to effectuate this right and it certainly may not intrude upon this right;

2) the constitutional right to make and have carried out

LSMT decisions is not limited (and could not be limited under the Fourteenth Amendment's equal protection clause) to terminally ill or PVS patients;

3) there is no meaningful legal distinction between withdrawing treatment and withholding its initiation in the first place; and

4) there is no meaningful legal distinction between decisions concerning artificial feeding tubes and other forms of LSMT.

Thus, state statutes that limit patient autonomy concerning LSMT decisions are subject to constitutional challenge and judicial invalidation, as has occurred in the several cases to date in which the issue has been raised.[12,13,14]

The big problem, however, is that physicians and other health care professionals, quite understandably, do not usually comprehend and act upon the law in the same way that sophisticated appellate judges and law professors do. Instead, misperceptions of legal requirements that feed into their natural risk-averse predilections (at least when it comes to their own legal exposure)[15]—often fueled by the overly conservative advice supplied by inhouse counsel[16] and risk managers[17]—frequently cause physicians to follow the path of apparent least resistance, even at the expense of patient and family autonomy and their own ethical and clinical preferences. To many physicians, the advance directive and/or family consent statutes on the books in their particular jurisdiction, however restrictive and counterproductive, represent the applicable law on LSMT decision-making. Astute lectures explaining how these statutes fit with and supplement, rather than supplant, constitutional and common law[18] rights may have little impact on medical behavior.

Threat of Litigation

Where the law is (or appears to be) uncertain and unpredictable, litigation is likely to be stirred up excessively. Par-

ties befuddled about their rights, responsibilities, and potential liabilities are much more likely to seek advance
judicial imprimature for their acts, even if all the parties
agree informally. State statutes that, by creating confusion
through inconsistency with other sources of law or by virtually inviting families to litigate,[19] increase formal resort
to the courts, turn precisely on its head the humane, sensible preference widely accepted in legal, ethical, and clinical
circles for private decisionmaking based on communication and negotiation. In doing so, restrictive state laws
sorely defeat the very purpose of advance directives, which
is to keep LSMT decisionmaking away from the judicial
system, except in very clear situations of egregious and
harmful conflicts of interest between the patient and
others.

Excessive litigation over LSMT decisions is expensive,
time-consuming, and emotionally draining. It also fans the
flames of disharmony and adversariness among patient,
family (often within the family), and health care providers
at precisely the time that trust, compassion, and unity
should prevail.

Discouragement of Time-Limited Trials

Another serious problem with unduly restrictive state
advance directive and family consent legislation is that
time-limited trials of potentially beneficial treatments will
be discouraged. Often, it is impossible to predict prospectively which critically ill patients may benefit from specific
medical interventions. Our public policies should encourage time-limited trials of treatments for patients in the
"gray zone," with everyone involved knowing that the treatment decision may be reassessed and that, if desired, the
treatment may subsequently be discontinued. However,
state statutes that, on their face or in their interpretation,
restrict the participants' options for withdrawal of treatment will probably frighten some patients, families, and
physicians into foregoing many treatments completely,

rather than risk the life sentence on machinery threatened by state statute. Some patients for whom treatment thus is foregone will suffer as a result.

Suicide

Some patients may be so traumatized by the vision of a future in which, despite their best in advance planning and forthright communication, certain nontreatment options are discouraged by restrictive state statutes, that they may even be motivated to act prematurely and commit suicide, seeing it as the only apparent way to control their own destinies. Restrictive state statutes, rather than protecting vulnerable patients, may inspire the specter of more Janet Adkins-type patients, contemplating long periods of extreme and irreversible mental decline and suffering prior to becoming terminally ill or PVS, and collaborating with more Dr. Kevorkians in "suicide machine" scenarios rather than serving as prisoners of a reluctant but risk management-bound medical system.

Distributive Justice

State statutes that impinge on LSMT decisionmaking autonomy violate the fundamental ethical principle of social or distributive justice. They waste scarce resources that could be put to good use in providing access to needed and desired services for those currently outside the health care system. Whether potentially beneficial medical treatments should be expressly rationed for certain patients without their consent, in order to conserve resources for competing uses, is an important issue, but one beyond the scope of this chapter. What is certain, though, is that state advance directive statutes that, in effect, force patients to endure expensive medical interventions that they or their surrogates believe fail to contribute to the quality of life harm not only the physical and emotional integrity and dignity of the patient, but also the well-being of others, for whom the resources now inappropriately and involuntarily consumed could be used beneficially. For example, how many people who now are without ready access to appropriate health services might benefit measurably from redirecting some of the extensive resources presently being pre-empted by an Ohio patient without an advance directive, lying in a persistent unconscious state for a year before the family is empowered to seek a court order to withdraw treatment?

Disrespect for the Law

Finally, state advance directive and family consent statutes that violate basic principles of patient and family autonomy and beneficence, sound clinical judgment, social or distributive justice, and the ethical standards of the health professions to "do no harm" probably will encourage public and professional disrespect for the law and even quiet but widespread civil disobedience. State-provoked disrespect for and violation of the law, especially in matters as essential as life and death, bode poorly for the long-range health of a democratic society.

PRACTICAL GUIDELINES FOR PHYSICIANS

In the wake of unduly restrictive state advance directive and family consent legislation, how should the physician react who is committed to humane and respectful care of the critically ill? Openly defying the law is not an option unless one is willing to shoulder the liability risks that attach to such conduct. However, in evaluating alternatives, the physician should consult with legal counsel for the physician's institution and with the risk manager for the institution to get a comprehensive and reasonable interpretation of the applicable law in his or her jurisdiction that takes into account constitutional and common law sources as well as the state statute.

Constitutional law consists of the text and judicial interpretations of the text of the basic organizational document of a government. Both the federal and individual state constitutions contain an enumeration of rights that individuals enjoy to protect them against unreasonable governmental interference. Neither statutes nor common law decisions are allowed to violate constitutional protections in the American system of democracy.

Statutes are laws enacted by elected legislative bodies on the basis of authority granted to the legislature by the government's constitution, and legislative activity may not exceed that grant of authority. Common law is judge-made precedent established through an evolutionary process of courts adjudicating claims that are litigated on a case-by-case basis. Thus, "the Law" is not a monolithic, self-contained entity, but instead a complex, multiheaded creature. One's state statute is just a single piece of the legal puzzle, and one that is influenced and constrained in effect by other sources of legal authority. Legal and risk management counsel should reflect and explain this complexity.

Actual legal risks of civil or criminal liability should be placed in a realistic perspective, taking into consideration the manner in which the legal and health care systems operate in fact.[20] Legal and risk management advice that seems irrational on its face may well be so and ought, at least, to be probed. Multiple opinions may be worthwhile.

Frank discussions should be conducted among patient, physician, and family as early as possible in the relationship regarding mutual agreeable principles of LMST decisionmaking. The physician should share with the patient and family his or her own philosophy and relevant religious and moral convictions that might affect the patient's care. The patient should be counseled concerning any interpretation of state advance directive or family consent statutes that the physician believes precludes him or her from honoring patient choices, so that an appropriate transfer to another physician can be attempted if desired. Just as patients (with physician encouragement) should communicate preferences to the physician, a timely reciprocal exchange of views about both personal philosophy and the felt limits of the law ought to occur. The ideal time for such an exchange is well before a crisis has arisen, which is prior to the point that the PSDA formally mandates provider action in this regard.

Although both the PSDA and most state statutes place a great deal of weight on the creation and transmission of written documents, and those pieces of paper are important in demonstrating compliance with the minimum letter of the law, the documents are not a substitute for personal conversation. The paperwork associated with advance health care planning should be considered an adjunct and stimulus to physician/patient/family interaction, rather than an excuse for avoiding it. The supplementary use of formal or informal tools for sharing values is by no means precluded by existing legislation.

The PSDA permits states to use consortia to help draft descriptions of state policies on medical decisionmaking. Physicians in California joined with over 20 other professional and consumer groups to produce a brochure and videotape to inform patients of their right to participate in medical decisions, including the formulation of advance directives. This grass-roots cooperation should be and, to a certain extent, is being emulated elsewhere.

Ultimately, if physicians agree with this author's objections to restrictive state advance directive and family consent statutes, and believe that many of the substantive and procedural barriers to choice erected by these statutes are an affront not only to patients and families but to the ethical and clinical integrity of the medical profession, they must exert efforts both individually and collectively, through pertinent professional associations, to bring about statutory modification. Several examples of desirable state legislation, such as the Virginia and District of Columbia family consent provisions, may be suggested as models. Legislative improvement may be accomplished by educating and lobbying state legislatures and regulatory agencies about the actual consequences of their public policies, using data systematically gathered in the course of clinical practice about the impact of the statutes on the lives of real patients and families. If may also be necessary in extreme situations to support patients and their families in bringing court challenges, asserting constitutional and common law guarantees of individual rights against the intrusion of the state into the most intimate of human affairs.

REFERENCES

1. Cruzan v. Director, Missouri Department Health 110 S.Ct. 2841 (1990).

2. McCloskey, E.L. Bioethics inside the beltway: The Patient Self-Determination Act. Kennedy Inst Ethics J 1991: 163–169.

3. Public Law 101–508, Sections 4206 (Medicare) and 4751 (Medicaid), 104 Stat. 1388.

4. LaPuma, J., Orentlicher, D., Moss, R.J. Advance directives on admission: Clinical implications of the Patient Self-Determination Act of 1990. JAMA 1991:266:402–405.

5. *Choice in dying, Refusal of Treatment Legislation*. New York: Author. 1991.

6. Ohio Amended Substitute Senate Bill No. 1 (1991).

7. Areen, J. Advance directives under state law and judicial decisions. Law Med Health Care 1991:19.

8. *Ibid.*, pp. 91–100.

9. Rouse, F. The role of state legislatures after Cruzan: What can—and should—state legislatures do? Law Med Health Care 1991:19:83–90.

10. Meisel, A. Legal myths about terminating life support. Arch Intern Med 1991:151:1497–1302.

11. Orentlicher, D. The right to die after Cruzan, JAMA 1990:264:2444–2446.

12. McConnell v. Beverly Enterprises, 209 Conn 892. 353 A.2d 596(1989).

13. In re Browning, 543 So.2d 258 (Fla.Dist.Ct. App. 1989), aff'd, 568 So.2d 4.

14. Corbett v. D'Alessandro, 487 So.2d 368 (Fla. Dist. Ct. App.), rev. denied. 492 So. 2d 1331 (Fla. 1986)

15. Kapp, M.B. Our hands are tied; Legally induced moral tensions in health care delivery. J Gen Inter Med 1009:6:345–348

16. Family privacy and persistent vegetative state; A symposium on the Linares case. Law Med Health Care 1989:17:295–346.

17. Kapp, M.B. Are risk management and health care ethics compatible? Perspectives in Healthcare Risk Management 1991 (Winter) 11:2–7.

18. Wolf, S. Honoring broader directives. Hastings Cent Rep 1991 (Sept–Oct); 21:S8–S9.

19. In re Estate of Longway, 133 Ill.2d. 33, 549 NE2d 292 (1989).

20. Kapp, M.B., Lo, B. Legal perceptions and medical decision making. Milbank Q 1986:64 (Supplement 2): 163–202.

Appendices

Appendix I

SELECTED LAWS

1. Text of the Patient Self-Determination Act

Omnibus Budget Reconciliation Act of 1990
P.L. 101-508

SEC. 4206. MEDICARE PROVIDER AGREEMENTS ASSURING THE IMPLEMENTATION OF A PATIENT'S RIGHT TO PARTICIPATE IN AND DIRECT HEALTH CARE DECISIONS AFFECTING THE PATIENT.
(a) In General.—Section 1866 (a)(1) (42 U.S.C. 1395cc(a)(1) is amended—

(1) in subsection (a)(1)—

(A) by striking "and" at the end of subparagraph (O).

(B) by striking the period at the end of subparagraph (P) and inserting ", and". and

(C) by inserting after subparagraph (P) the following new subparagraph:

"(Q) in the case of hospitals, skilled nursing facilities, home health agencies and hospice programs, to

comply with the requirement of subsection (f) (relating
to maintaining written policies and procedures
respecting advance directives).''; and

(2) by inserting after subsection (e) the following new
subsection:

''(f)(1) For purposes of subsection (a)(1)(Q) and sections
1819 (c)(2)(E), 1833(r), 1876(c)(8), and 1891(a)(6), the
requirement of this subsection is that a provider of
services or prepaid or eligible organization (as the case
may be) maintain written policies and procedures with
respect to all adult individuals receiving medical care by
or through the provider or organization—

''(A) to provide written information to each such
individual concerning—

''(i) an individual's rights under State law (whether
statutory or as recognized by the courts of the State)
to make decisions concerning such medical care,
including the right to accept or refuse medical or
surgical treatment and the right to formulate advance
directives (as defined in paragraph (3)), and

''(ii) the written policies of the provider or
organization respecting the implementation of such
rights;

''(B) to document in the individual's medical record
whether or not the individual has executed an advance
directive;

''(C) not to condition the provision of care or otherwise
discriminate against an individual based on whether
or not the individual has executed an advance
directive;

''(D) to ensure compliance with requirements of State
law (whether statutory or as recognized by the courts
of the State) respecting advance directives at facilities
of the provider or organization; and

"(E) to provide (individually or with others) for education for staff and the community on issues concerning advance directives.

Subparagraph (C) shall not be construed as requiring the provision of care which conflicts with an advance directive.

"(2) The written information described in paragraph (1) (A) shall be provided to an adult individual—

"(A) in the case of a hospital, at the time of the individual's admission as an inpatient,

"(B) in the case of a skilled nursing facility, at the time of the individual's admission as a resident,

"(C) in the case of a home health agency, in advance of the individual coming under the care of the agency,

"(D) in the case of a hospice program, at the time of initial receipt of hospice care by the individual from the program, and

"(E) in the case of an eligible organization (as defined in section 1876 (b)) or an organization provided payments under section 1833(a)(1)(A), at the time of enrollment of the individual with the organization.

"(3) In this subsection, the term 'advance directive' means a written instruction, such as a living will or durable power of attorney for health care, recognized under State law (whether statutory or as recognized by the courts of the State) and relating to the provision of such care when the individual is incapacitated.".

(b) Application to Prepaid Organizations.—(1) Eligible Organizations.—Section 1876(c) of such Act (42 U.S C. 1395mm(c)) is amended by adding at the end the following new paragraph:

"(8) A contract under this section shall provide that the

eligible organization shall meet the requirement of section 1866 (f) (relating to maintaining written policies and procedures respecting advance directives)."

(2) Other Prepaid Organizations.—Section 1833 of such Act (42 U.S.C. 13951) is amended by adding at the end the following new subsection:

"(r) The Secretary may not provide for payment under subsection (a) (1) (A) with respect to an organization unless the organization provides assurances satisfactory to the Secretary that the organization meets the requirement of section 1866 (f) (relating to maintaining written policies and procedures respecting advance directives).".

(c) Effect on State Law.—Nothing in subsections (a) and (b) shall be construed to prohibit the application of a State law which allows for an objection on the basis of conscience for any health care provider or any agent of such provider which, as a matter of conscience, cannot implement an advance directive.

(d) Conforming Amendments.—

(1) Section 1819 (c) (1) of such Act (42 U.S.C. 1395i-3(c) (1)) is amended by adding at the end the following new subparagraph:

"(E) Information Respecting Advance Directives.—A skilled nursing facility must comply with the requirement of section 1866(f) (relating to maintaining written policies and procedures respecting advance directives).".

(2) Section 1891(a) of such Act (42 U.S.C. 1395bbb(a)) is amended by adding at the end the following:

"(6) The agency complies with the requirement of section 1866 (f) (relating to maintaining written policies and procedures respecting advance directives).".

(e) Effective Dates.—

(1) The amendments made by subsections (a) and (d) shall apply with respect to services furnished on or after the first day of the first month beginning more than 1 year after the date of the enactment of this Act.

(2) The amendments made by subsection (b) shall apply to contracts under section 1876 of the Social Security Act and payments under section 1833 (a)(1)(A) of such Act on the first day of the first month beginning more than 1 year after the date of the enactment of this Act.

SEC. 4751. REQUIREMENTS FOR ADVANCED DIRECTIVES UNDER STATE PLANS FOR MEDICAL ASSISTANCE.

(a) In General.—Section 1902 (42 U.S.C. 1396a(a)), as amended by sections 4401(a)(2), 4601(d), 4701(a), 4711, and 4722 of this title, is amended—

(1) in subsection (a)—

(A) by striking "and" at the end of paragraph (55).

(B) by striking the period at the end of paragraph (56) and inserting "; and", and

(C) by inserting after paragraph (56) the following new paragraphs:

"(57) provide that each hospital, nursing facility, provider of home health care or personal care services, hospice program, or health maintenance organization (as defined in section 1903(m)(1)(A)) receiving funds under the plan shall comply with the requirements of subsection (w):

"(58) provide that the State, acting through a State agency, association, or other private nonprofit entity, develop a written description of the law of the State (whether statutory or as recognized by the courts of the

State) concerning advance directives that would be distributed by providers or organizations under the requirements of subsection (w).''; and

(2) by adding at the end the following new subsection:

''(w)(1) For purposes of subsection (a)(57) and sections 1903 (m)(1)(a) and 1919 (c)(2)(E), the requirement of this subsection is that a provider or organization (as the case may be) maintain written policies and procedures with respect to all adult individuals receiving medical care by or through the provider or organization—

(A) to provide written information to each such individual concerning—

''(i) an individual's rights under State law (whether statutory or as recognized by the courts of the State) to make decisions concerning such medical care, including the right to accept or refuse medical or surgical treatment and the right to formulate advance directives (as defined in paragraph (3)), and

''(ii) the provider's or organization's written policies respecting the implementation of such rights;

''(B) to document in the individual's medical record whether or not the individual has executed an advance directive;

''(C) not to condition the provision of care or otherwise discriminate against an individual based on whether or not the individual has executed an advance directive;

''(D) to ensure compliance with requirements of State law (whether statutory or as recognized by the courts of the State) respecting advance directives; and

''(E) to provide (individually or with others) for education for staff and the community on issues concerning advance directives.

Subparagraph (C) shall not be construed as requiring the

provision of care which conflicts with an advance directive.

"(2) The written information described in paragraph (1)(A) shall be provided to an adult individual—

"(A) in the case of a hospital, at the time of the individual's admission as an inpatient.

"(B) in the case of a nursing facility, at the time of the individual's admission as a resident,

"(C) in the case of a provider of home health care or personal care services, in advance of the individual coming under the care of the provider.

"(D) in the case of a hospice program, at the time of initial receipt of hospice care by the individual from the program, and

"(E) in the case of a health maintenance organization, at the time of enrollment of the individual with the organization.

"(3) Nothing in this section shall be construed to prohibit the application of a State law which allows for an objection on the basis of conscience for any health care provider or any agent of such provider which as a matter of conscience cannot implement an advance directive."

"(4) In this subsection, the term 'advance directive' means a written instruction, such as a living will or durable power of attorney for health care, recognized under State law whether statutory or as recognized by the courts of the State and relating to the provision of such care when the individual is incapacitated.

(b) Conforming Amendments.—

(1) section 1903(m)(1)(A)(42 U.S.C. 1396b(m)(1)(A) is amended—

(A) by inserting "meets the requirement of section

1902 (w)" after "which" the first place it appears
and

(B) by inserting "meets the requirement of section
1902(a) and" after "which" the second place it
appears.

(2) Section 1919 (c)(2) of such Act (42 U.S.C. 1396r(c)(2))
is amended by adding at the end the following new
subparagraph:

"(E) Information respecting advance directives.—A
nursing facility must comply with the requirement
of section 1902(w) (relating to maintaining written
policies and procedures respecting advance
directives).".

(c) Effective Date.—The amendments made by this
section shall apply with respect to services furnished on
or after the first day of the first month beginning more
than 1 year after the date of the enactment of this Act.

(d) Public Education Campaign.—

(1) In General.—The Secretary, no later than 6 months
after the date of enactment of this section, shall
develop and implement a national campaign to inform
the public of the option to execute advance directives
and of a patient's rights to participate and direct
health care decisions.

(2) Development and Distribution of Information.—The
Secretary shall develop or approve nationwide
informational materials that would be distributed by
providers under the requirements of this section, to
inform the public and the medical and legal profession
of each person's right to make decisions concerning
medical care, including the right to accept or refuse
medical or surgical treatment, and the existence of
advance directives.

(3) Providing Assistance to States.—The Secretary shall
assist appropriate State agencies, associations, or

other private entities in developing the State-specific documents that would be distributed by providers under the requirements of this section. The Secretary shall further assist appropriate State agencies, associations, or other private entities in ensuring that providers are provided a copy of the documents that are to be distributed under the requirements of the section.

(4) Duties of Secretary.—The Secretary shall mail information to Social Security recipients, add a page to the medicare handbook with respect to the provisions of this section.

2. State Statutes

Alabama Natural Death Act, Ala. Code §§ 22-8A-1 to -10 (1990)
Alabama Durable Power of Attorney Act, Ala. Code §§ 26-1-2 (1986)
Alaska Rights of Terminally Ill Act, Alaska Stat. 18.12.010 to -.100 (Supp. 1990)
Alaska Statutory Form Power of Attorney Act, Alaska Stat. §§ 13.26.332 to 13.26.353 (Supp. 1990)
Arizona Living Wills and Health Care Directives Act, Ariz. Rev. Stat. Ann. §§ 36-3201 to -3261
Arkansas Rights of the Terminally Ill or Permanently Unconscious Act, Ark. Code Ann. §§ 20-17-201 to -218 (Supp. 1989)
Arkansas Durable Power of Attorney Act, Ark. Code Ann. §§ 28-68-201 to -203 (1987)
California Natural Death Act, Cal. Health & Safety Code §§ 7185 to 7194.5 (West Supp. 1992)
California Durable Power of Attorney for Health Care Act, Cal. Civil Code §§ 2430 to 2444 (West Supp. 1992)
California Statutory Form Durable Power of Attorney for Health Care Act, Cal. Civil Code §§ 2500 to 2508 (West Supp. 1992)
Colorado Medical Treatment Decision Act, Colo. Rev. Stat. §§ 15-18-101 to -113 (1987 & Supp. 1991)
Colorado Patient Autonomy Act, Colo. Rev. Stat. §§ 15-14-501 to -509 (S.B. 3, 1992)
Connecticut Removal of Life Support Systems Act, Conn. Gen. Stat. §§ 19a-570 to -580 (1993)

Connecticut Statutory Short Form Durable Power of Attorney
    Act, Conn. Gen. Stat. §§ 1-43 to -54a (Supp. 1991 & Pub. Act
    91-382) (1991)
Delaware Death with Dignity Act, Del. Code Ann. tit. 16, §§ 2501
    to 2509 (1983)
Delaware Uniform Durable Power of Attorney Act, Del. Code Ann.,
    tit. 12, §§ 4901-4905 (1987)
District of Columbia Natural Death Act of 1981, D.C. Code Ann. §§
    6-2421 to -2430 (1989)
District of Columbia Health-Care Decisions Act of 1988, D.C. Code
    Ann. §§ 21-2201 to -2213 (1989)
Florida Health Care Advance Directives Act, Fla. Stat. Ann. §§
    765.101 to -.113; 765.201 to -.205; 765.301 to -.310; 765.401
    (1992)
Georgia Living Wills Act, Ga. Code Ann. §§ 31-32-1 to -12 (Michie
    1991 & H.B. 968, 1992)
Georgia Durable Power of Attorney for Health Care Act, Ga. Code
    §§ 31-36-1 to -13 (Michie 1991)
Georgia Orders Not to Resuscitate Act (S.B. 93, 1991)
Hawaii Medical Treatment Decisions Act, Hawaii Rev. Stat. §§
    327D-1 to -27 (Supp. 1991)
Hawaii Uniform Durable Power of Attorney, for Health Care Deci-
    sions Act, Hawaii Rev. Stat. § 551D (H.B. 1930, 1992)
Idaho Natural Death Act, Idaho Code §§ 39-4501 to -4509 (1985 &
    Supp. 1989)
Illinois Living Will Act, Ill. Ann. Stat. ch. 110 1/2 §§ 701 to 710
    (Smith-Hurd Supp. 1991)
Illinois Powers of Attorney for Health Care Act, Ill. Ann. Stat. ch.
    110 1/2, §§ 804-1 to -11 (Smith-Hurd Supp. 1991)
Illinois Health Care Surrogate Act, H.B. 2334 (1991)
Indiana Living Wills and Life-Prolonging Procedures Act, Ind.
    Code Ann. §§ 16-8-11-1 to -22 (Burns 1990)
Indiana Powers of Attorney Act, Ind. Code Ann. §§ 30-5-1-1 to 10-4
    (Supp. 1991)
Indiana Health Care Consent Act, Ind. Code Ann. §§ 16-8-12-2
    (1990), as interpreted by In re Lawrence, No. 29504-9106-CV-
    00460 (Ind. Sept. 17, 1991)
Iowa Life-Sustaining Procedures Act, Iowa Code Ann. §§ 144A.1 to
    -.11 (1989 & H.F. 2207, 1992)
Iowa Durable Power of Attorney for Health Care Act, Iowa Code
    Ann. §§ 144B.1 to -.12 (Supp. 1992)

Kansas Natural Death Act, Kan. Stat. Ann. §§ 65-28, 101 to -28,109 (1985)

Kansas Durable Power of Attorney for Health Care Decisions Act, Kan. Stat. Ann. §§ 58-625 to -632 (Supp. 1989)

Kentucky Living Will Act, Ky. Rev. Stat. §§ 311.622 to -.642 (Supp. 1990)

Kentucky Health Care Surrogate Act, Ky. Rev. Stat. §§ 311.970 to -.986 (Supp. 1990)

Louisiana Life-Sustaining Procedures Act, La. Rev. Stat. Ann. 40:1299.58.1 to -.10 (Supp. 1991 & H.B. 275, 1991 & S.B. 532, S.B. 540 & S.B. 723, 1991)

Louisiana Power of Attorney Act, No. 184 (H.B. 713, 1990) and Life-Sustaining Procedures Act, § 1299.58.5A(2) (a)

Maine Uniform Rights of the Terminally Ill Act, Me. Rev. Stat. Ann. tit. 18-A, §§ 5-701 to -714 (West Supp. 1991)

Maine Powers of Attorney Act, Me. Rev. Stat. Ann. tit. 18-A, §§ 5-501 to -502 (West Supp. 1991)

Maryland Life-Sustaining Procedures Act, Md. Health-General Code Ann. §§ 5-601 to -614 (Supp. 1988)

Maryland Durable Power of Attorney Act, Md. Est. & Trust Code Ann. §§ 13-601 to -603 (1974), as interpreted by 73 Opinions of the Attorney General _____ [Opinion No. 88-046 (October 17, 1988)]; 75 Opinions of the Attorney General _____ (1990) [Opinion No. 90-044 (September 24, 1990)]

Massachusetts Health Care Proxies by Individuals Act, Mass. Gen. L. ch. 201D (Supp. 1991)

Michigan Power of Attorney for Health Care Act, Mich. Comp. Law, §§ 700.496 (West Supp. 1992)

Minnesota Adult Health Care Decisions Act, Minn. Stat. §§ 145B.01 to -.17 (Supp. 1992 & S.F. 2111, 1992)

Minnesota Statutory Short Form Durable Power of Attorney Act, Minn. Stat. §§ 523.01 to -.25 (1988)

Mississippi Withdrawal of Life-Saving Mechanisms Act, Miss. Code Ann. §§ 41-41-101 to -121 (Supp. 1988)

Mississippi Durable Power of Attorney for Health Care Act, Miss. Code Ann. §§ 41-41-151 to -183 (Supp. 1990)

Missouri Life Support Declarations Act, Mo. Ann. Stat. §§ 459.010 to -.055 (Vernon Supp. 1992)

Missouri Durable Power of Attorney for Health Care Act, Mo. Ann. Stat. §§ 404.800 to -.870 (Vernon Supp. 1992)

Montana Rights of the Terminally Ill Act, Mont. Code Ann. §§ 50-9-101 to -111, -201 to -206 (1991)

Montana Durable Power of Attorney Act, Mont. Code Ann. §§ 72-5-501 to -502 (1991)

Montana Do Not Resuscitate Notification Act, Mont. Health and Safety §§ 50-10-101 to 50-10-106 (1991)

Nebraska Rights of the Terminally Ill Act, L.B. 671 (1992)

Nebraska Power of Attorney for Health Care Act, L.B. 696 (1992)

Nevada Uniform Act on the Rights of the Terminally Ill, Nev. Rev. Stat. §§ 449.535 to -.690 (1991)

Nevada Durable Power of Attorney for Health Care Act, Nev. Rev. Stat. Ann. §§ 449.800 to -.860 (1991)

New Hampshire Living Wills Act, N.H. Rev. Stat. Ann. §§ 137-H:1-H:16 (Supp. 1991 & H.B. 1108, 1992)

New Hampshire Durable Power of Attorney for Health Care, N.H. Rev. Stat. Ann. §§ 137-J:1 to -J:16 (Supp. 1991)

New Jersey Advance Directives for Health Care Act, N.J. Stat. Ann. §§ 26:2H-53 to -78 (West Supp. 1992)

New Mexico Right to Die Act, N.M. Stat. Ann. §§ 24-7-1 to -11 (1986)

New Mexico Durable Power of Attorney Act, N.M. Stat. Ann. §§ 45-5-501 to -502 (Supp. 1989)

New York Health Care Proxy Act, N.Y. Pub. Health Law §§ 2980 to 2994 (McKinney Supp. 1991)

New York Orders Not to Resuscitate Act, N.Y. Pub. Health Law §§ 2960-2978 (McKinney 1989 & A. 7429, 1991)

North Carolina Right to Natural Death Act, N.C. Gen. Stat. §§ 90-320 to -322 (Supp. 1991)

North Carolina Health Care Powers of Attorney Act, N.C. Gen. Stat. §§ 32A-15 to -26 (1991)

North Dakota Uniform Rights of the Terminally Ill Act, N.D. Cent. Code §§ 23-06.4-01 to -14 (Supp. 1989 & Interim Supp. 1991)

North Dakota Durable Powers of Attorney for Health Care Act, N.D. Cent. Stat. §§ 23-06.5-01 to -18 (Interim Supp. 1991)

Ohio Modified Uniform Rights of the Terminally Ill Act, Ohio Rev. Code Ann. §§ 2133.01 to -.15 (Anderson Supp. 1991)

Ohio Power of Attorney Act for Health Care, Ohio Rev. Code Ann. §§ 1337.11 to -.17 (Anderson Supp. 1991)

Oklahoma Rights of the Terminally Ill or Persistently Unconscious Act, Okla. Stat. Ann. tit. 63, §§ 3101.1 to -.16 (H.B. 1893, 1992)

Oklahoma Hydration & Nutrition for Incompetent Patients Act, Okla. Stat. Ann. tit. 63, §§ 3080.1 to -.5 (Supp. 1992 & H.B. 1893, 1992)

Oregon Rights with Respect to Terminal Illness Act, Or. Rev. Stat. §§ 127.605 to -.650 (1990)

Oregon Durable Power of Attorney for Health Care Act, Or. Rev. Stat. §§ 127.505 to -.585 (1990)

Oregon Patient Self-Determination Act, S.B. 787 (1991)

Pennsylvania Advance Directive for Health Care Act, Pa. Stat. Ann. tit. 20, §§ 5401-5416 (S.B. 3, 1992)

Rhode Island Rights of the Terminally Ill Act, R.I. Gen. Laws §§ 23-4.11 to -.13 (Supp. 1991 & H.B. 9037, 1992)

Rhode Island Health Care Power of Attorney Act, R.I. Gen. Laws 23-4.10-1 to -2 (1989 & H.B. 9037, 1992)

South Carolina Death with Dignity Act, S.C. Code Ann. §§ 44-77-10 to -160 (Law. Co-Op Supp. 1991)

South Carolina Powers of Attorney Act, S.C. Code Ann. §§ 62-5-501 to -504 (Law. Co-Op Supp. 1991 & S.B. 510, 1992 & S.B. 541, 1992)

South Carolina Adult Health Care Consent Act, S.C. Code Ann. §§ 44-66-10 to -80 (Law. Co-Op Supp. 1991 & S.B. 541, 1992)

South Dakota Living Will Act, S.D. Codified Laws Ann. §§ 34-120-1-22 (Supp. 1991)

South Dakota Durable Powers of Attorney Act, S.D. Codified Laws Ann. §§ 59-7-2.1 to -2.8 (Supp. 1991 & H.B. 1131, 1992)

Tennessee Right to Natural Death Act, Tenn. Code Ann. §§ 32-11-101 to -112 (Supp. 1991)

Tennessee Durable Power of Attorney for Health Care Act, Tenn. Code Ann. §§ 34-6-101 to -214 (1991)

Texas Natural Death Act, Tex. Health & Safety Code Ann. §§ 672.001 to -.021 (1992)

Texas Durable Power of Attorney for Health Care Act, Tex. Civil Practice & Remedies Code Ann. §§ 135.001 to -.018 (Vernon Supp. 1992)

Utah Personal Choice and Living Will Act, Utah Code Ann. §§ 75-2-1101 to -1118 (Supp. 1990)

Utah Powers of Attorney Act, Utah Code Ann. §§ 75-5-501 to §§ -502 (1978)

Vermont Terminal Care Document Act, Vt. Stat. Ann. tit. 18, §§
    5251 to 5262 and tit. 13, § 1801 (1987)
Vermont Durable Power of Attorney for Health Care, Vt. Stat.
    Ann. tie. 14, ch. 121, §§ 3451 to 3467 (Supp. 1988)
Virginia Health Care Decisions Act, Va. Code §§ 54.1-2981 to -2993
    (S.B. 360, 1992, S.B. 254 & H.B. 819, 1992)
Virginia Substituted Consent Act, Va. Code § 37.1-134.4 (Supp.
    1991)
Virginia Durable Power of Attorney Act, Va. Code §§ 11-9.1 to -9.4
    (1989)
Washington Natural Death Act, Wash. Rev. Code Ann. §§
    70.122.010 to -.905 (Supp. 1991 & H.B. 1481, 1992)
Washington Durable Power of Attorney-Health Care Decisions
    Act, Wash. Rev. Code Ann. § 11.94.010 (Supp. 1991)
West Virginia Natural Death Act, W. Va. Code §§ 16-30-1 to -10
    (1985 & Supp. 1991)
West Virginia Medical Power of Attorney Act, W. Va. Code §§ 16-
    30a-1 to -20 (Supp. 1990)
Wisconsin Natural Death Act, Wisc. Stat. Ann. §§ 154.01 to -.15
    (West 1989 & Pub. Act 84 A.B. 559, 1991 & Pub. Act 281 S.B.
    415, 1992)
Wisconsin Power of Attorney for Health Care Act, Wisc. Stat. Ann.
    §§ 155.01 to -.80 (Supp. 1991 & Pub. Act. 281 S.B. 415, 1992)
Wyoming Living Will Act, Wyo. Stat., §§ 35-22-101 to -109 (1987 &
    Supp. 1991 & H.B. 24, 1992)
Wyoming Durable Power of Attorney for Health Care Act, Wyo.
    Stat., §§ 3-5-201 to -214 (Supp. 1991 & H.B. 24, 1992)

Appendix II

SELECTED ORGANIZATIONAL RESOURCES

American Academy of Medical Directors, 5205 Leesburg Pike, Falls Church, VA 22041

American Association of Homes for the Aging, 1129 20th Street, NW, Washington, DC 20036

American Association of Nurse Attorneys, 720 Light Street, Baltimore, MD 21230-3826

American Association of Retired Persons, 601 E Street, NW, Washington, DC 20049

American Bar Association, Commission on Legal Problems of the Elderly, 1800 M Street, NW, Washington, DC 20036

American Geriatrics Society, 770 Lexington Avenue, New York, NY 10021

American Health Care Association, 1201 L Street, NW, Washington, DC 20005

American Medical Directors Association, 10480 Little Patuxent Parkway, Suite 760, Columbia, MD 21044

American Society on Aging, 833 Market Street, San Francisco, CA 94103

American Society of Law, Medicine & Ethics, 765 Commonwealth Avenue, 16th Floor, Boston, MA 02215

Bioethics Consultation Group, 2322 Sixth Street, Berkeley, CA 94710

Catholic Health Association, 4455 Woodson Road, St. Louis, MO 63134

Center for Social Gerontology, 2307 Shelby Avenue, Ann Arbor,
    MI 48103-3895
Choice in Dying, 250 West 57th Street, New York, NY 10019
Dorothy Garske Center, 4250 East Camelback Road, Suite 185K,
    Phoenix, AZ 85018
Education Development Center, 55 Chapel Street, Newton, MA
    02160
Gerontological Society of America, 1411 K Street, NW, Washing-
    ton, DC 20005
Hastings Center, 255 Elm Road, Briarcliff Manor, NY 10510
Hemlock Society, P.O. Box 11830, Eugene, OR 97440
Institute of Public Law, University of New Mexico, 1117 Stanford
    Drive, NE, Albuquerque, NM 87106
Kennedy Institute of Ethics, Georgetown University, 37th and P
    Streets, NW, Washington, DC 20057 (Includes National Ref-
    erence Center for Bioethics Literature)
Legal Counsel for the Elderly, 601 E Street, NW, Washington, DC
    20049
National Association for Home Care, 519 C Street, NE, Washing-
    ton, DC 20002-5809
National Citizens Coalition for Nursing Home Reform, 1424 16th
    Street, NW, Washington, DC 20036
National Health Lawyers Association, 1120 Connecticut Avenue,
    NW, Washington, DC 20036-3902
National Hospice Organization, 1901 N. Fort Meyer Drive,
    Arlington, VA 22209
National Legal Center for the Medically Dependent & Disabled,
    Inc., P.O. Box 1586, Terre Haute, IN 47808-1586
National Senior Citizens Law Center, 1052 W. 6th Street, Los An-
    geles, CA 90017
Older Women's League, 730 11th Street, NW, Suite 300, Washing-
    ton, DC 20001
Pacific Center of Health Policy and Ethics, 444 Law Center, Uni-
    versity of Southern California, Los Angeles, CA 90089
Park Ridge Center for the Study of Health, Faith, and Ethics, 676
    N. St. Clair, Suite 450, Chicago, IL 60611
Society for Health and Human Values, 6728 Old McLean Village
    Drive, McLean, VA 22101
Veterans Administration National Center for Clinical Ethics, De-
    partment of Veterans Affairs, Medical Center, White River
    Junction, VT 05001

Appendix III

VALUES HISTORY

This Values History form was developed by the University of New Mexico Center for Health Law and Ethics, Institute of Public Law, as a part of a National Values History Project sponsored by a grant from the Ittleson Foundation. This document is not copyrighted.

The Values History
SECTION 1

A. WRITTEN LEGAL DOCUMENTS

Have you written any of the following legal documents? _

If so, please complete the requested information.

Living Will
Date written: _____
Document location: _____
Comments: (e.g., any limitations, special requests, etc.) ___
_____
_____

Durable Power of Attorney
Date written: _____
Document location: _____
Comments: (e.g., whom have you named to be your decision
maker?) _____
_____
_____

Durable Power of Attorney for Health Care Decisions
Date written: _____
Document location: _____
Comments: (e.g., whom have you named to be your decision
maker?) _____
_____
_____

Organ Donations
Date written: _____
Document location: _____
Comments: (e.g., any limitations on which organs you
would like to donate?) _____
_____
_____

B. WISHES CONCERNING SPECIFIC MEDICAL PROCE- DURES

If you have ever expressed your wishes, either written or
orally, concerning any of the following medical procedures, please complete the requested information. If you
have not previously indicated your wishes on these procedures and would like to do so now, please complete
this information.

Organ Donation
To whom expressed: _____
If oral, when? _____
If written, when? _____
Document location: _____
Comments: _____

_____

_____

Kidney Dialysis
To whom expressed: _____
If oral, when? _____
If written, when? _____
Document location: _____
Comments: _____

_____

Cardiopulmonary Resuscitation (CPR)
To whom expressed: _____
If oral, when? _____
If written, when? _____
Document location: _____
Comments: _____

_____

Respirators
To whom expressed: _____
If oral, when? _____
If written, when? _____
Document location: _____
Comments: _____

_____

Artificial Nutrition
To whom expressed: _____
If oral, when? _____
If written, when? _____
Document location: _____
Comments: _____

_____

Artificial hydration
To whom expressed: _____
If oral, when? _____
If written, when? _____

Document location: _____

Comments: _____

_____

_____

C. GENERAL COMMENTS

Do you wish to make any general comments about the information you provided in this section? _____

_____

_____

SECTION 2

A. YOUR OVERALL ATTITUDE TOWARD YOUR HEALTH

1. How would you describe your current health status? If you currently have any medical problems, how would you describe them? _____

_____

_____

2. If you have current medical problems, in what ways, if any, do they affect your ability to function? _____

_____

_____

3. How do you feel about your current health status? __

_____

_____

4. How well are you able to meet the basic necessities of life—eating, food preparation, sleeping, personal hygiene, etc.? _____

_____

_____

5. Do you wish to make any general comments about your overall health? _____

_____

_____

B. YOUR PERCEPTION OF THE ROLE OF YOUR DOCTOR AND OTHER HEALTH CAREGIVERS

1. Do you like your doctors? _____

2. Do you trust your doctors? _____

3. Do you think your doctors should make the final decision concerning any treatment you might need? _____
_____

4. How do you relate to your caregivers, including nurses, therapists, chaplains, social workers, etc.? _____
_____

5. Do you wish to make any general comments about your doctor and other health caregivers? _____
_____

C. YOUR THOUGHTS ABOUT INDEPENDENCE AND CONTROL

1. How important is independence and self-sufficiency in your life? _____
_____

2. If you were to experience decreased physical and mental abilities, how would that affect your attitude toward independence and self-sufficiency? _____
_____

3. Do you wish to make any general comments about the value of independence and control in your life? _____
_____

D. YOUR PERSONAL RELATIONSHIPS

1. Do you expect that your friends, family and/or others will support your decisions regarding medical treatment you may need now or in the future? _____

_____

2. Have you made any arrangements for your family or friends to make medical treatment decisions on your behalf? If so, who has agreed to make decisions for you and in what circumstances?

_____

3. What, if any, unfinished business from the past are you concerned about (e.g., personal and family relationships, business and legal matters)? _____

_____

4. What role do your friends and family play in your life? _____

_____

5. Do you wish to make any general comments about the personal relationships in your life? _____

_____

E. YOUR OVERALL ATTITUDE TOWARD LIFE

1. What activities do you enjoy (e.g., hobbies, watching TV, etc.)? _____

_____

2. Are you happy to be alive? _____

_____

3. Do you feel that life is worth living? _____

_____

4. How satisfied are you with what you have achieved in your life? _____

_____

5. What makes you laugh/cry? _____

_____

6. What do you fear most? _____ What frightens or upsets you?

_____

7. What goals do you have for the future? _____

_____

8. Do you wish to make any general comments about your attitude toward life? _____

_____

_____

F. YOUR ATTITUDE TOWARD ILLNESS, DYING, AND DEATH

1. What will be important to you when you are dying (e.g., physical comfort, no pain, family members present, etc.)? _____

_____

2. Where would you prefer to die? _____

_____

3. What is your attitude toward death? _____

_____

4. How do you feel about the use of life-sustaining measures in the face of: terminal illness? _____

_____

permanent coma? _____

_____

irreversible chronic illness (e.g., Alzheimer's disease)? ____

5. Do you wish to make any general comments about your attitude toward illness, dying, and death? _____

_____

_____

G. YOUR RELIGIOUS BACKGROUND AND BELIEFS

1. What is your religious background? _____

_____

2. How do your religious beliefs affect your attitude toward serious or terminal illness? _____

_____

3. Does your attitude toward death find support in your religion? _____

_____

4. How does your faith community, church or synagogue view the role of prayer or religious sacraments in an illness? _____

_____

5. Do you wish to make any general comments about your religious background and beliefs? _____

_____

H. YOUR LIVING ENVIRONMENT

1. What has been your living situation over the last 10 years (e.g., lived alone, lived with others, etc.)? _____

_____

2. How difficult is it for you to maintain the kind of environment for yourself that you find comfortable? Does any

illness or medical problem you have now mean that it will be harder in the future?

_____

3. Do you wish to make any general comments about your living environment? _____

_____

I. YOUR ATTITUDE CONCERNING FINANCES

1. How much do you worry about having enough money to provide for your care? _____

_____

2. Would you prefer to spend less money on your care so that more money can be saved for the benefit of your relatives and/or friends? _____

_____

3. Do you wish to make any general comments concerning your finances and the cost of health care? _____

_____

J. YOUR WISHES CONCERNING YOUR FUNERAL

1. What are your wishes concerning your funeral and burial or cremation? _____

_____

_____

2. Have you made your funeral arrangements? If so, with whom?_____

_____

3. Do you wish to make any general comments about how you would like your funeral and burial or cremation to be arranged or conducted? _____

_____

_____

_____

_____

OPTIONAL QUESTIONS

1. How would you like your obituary (announcement of your death) to read? _____

_____

_____

_____

_____

2. Write yourself a brief eulogy (a statement about yourself to be read at your funeral). _____

_____

_____

_____

_____

SUGGESTIONS FOR USE

After you have completed this form, you may wish to provide copies to your doctors and other health caregivers, your family, your friends, and your attorney. If you have a Living Will or Durable Power of Attorney for Health Care Decisions, you may wish to attach a copy of this form to those documents.

Appendix IV

MODEL ADVANCE DIRECTIVE

"Instructions to My Surrogate" is a document developed by the Philadelphia Geriatric Center, 5301 Old York Road, Philadelphia, PA, and is reprinted here with the permission of the Philadelphia Geriatric Center.

Philadelphia Geriatric Center

ADVANCE MEDICAL DIRECTIVE

Introduction

Many people are concerned about their medical care if they become unable to make their own decisions because of poor physical or mental health. Although it is difficult to think about the situations which might occur as our health declines, taking time to think about our wishes in advance can ensure that decisions which will be made will be as we want them to be.

This packet includes three documents which can give you control over your medical care in the event that you are not able to make your own decisions. The documents are:

1) Durable Power of Attorney for Healthcare
   The Durable Power of Attorney for Health Care allows
   you to determine *who* will make medical decisions for
   you should you become unable to do so. In this document, you appoint this person, called a *surrogate*, and
   alternates, if you wish.

2) Living Will ("Pennsylvania Declaration")
   This document allows you to indicate your wishes
   about healthcare in specific circumstances: terminal
   illness, permanent unconsciousness (coma) or persis-
   tive vegetative state. Pennsylvania law makes these instructions *binding on your physician*.

3) Instructions to My Surrogate
   The advance medical directive statement, "Instructions to my Surrogate," provides you with a way to advise your surrogate decision-maker of your wishes, so
   that he or she can make decisions based on what you
   would want. These instructions are advisory and are
   not legally binding on your surrogate; he or she may
   judge situations as they arise. Of course, it is important that you discuss this document with your surrogate (and alternate surrogate) and your doctor.

It is your decision as to whether to complete these documents. You are free to use all, some or none of them. PGC
staff are available to help explain the documents to you, or
to help you to fill them out, if you wish.

Instructions to My Surrogate

I understand that I can make my own medical decisions as
long as I have the ability to do so. If I can no longer make
my own decisions, either permanently or temporarily, I ask
you, my surrogate, to use the following information to help
you in making decisions for me based on my values and
goals.

I. My Most Important Values
The most important things to me with respect to my health and healthcare are: (Check as many as you wish)

_____ To live as long as possible, even if my ability to function becomes impaired. (you may explain further)

_____

_____

_____ To maintain my dignity. (please explain further)

_____

_____

_____ To have a satisfying quality of life. (please explain further)

_____

_____

_____ To be able to communicate with other people. (you may explain further)

_____

_____

_____ To be free from pain. (you may explain further)

_____

_____

_____ Other (please specify)

_____

_____

II. Treatment Approaches

Many people have feelings about what kind of treatment they would want to receive in particular circumstances. This section allows you to give your surrogate general guidance for different situations which might occur in the event you become unable to decide for yourself.

In any given situation, there is a range of **treatment approaches**, ranging from *comfort care only* (in which treatments are used only for the purpose of alleviating pain and controlling symptoms) to *selective treatment* (in which prolonging life is weighed against the quality of life), and *maximum treatment* (designed to prolong life as long as possible).

Comfort care only: I would like **limited** treatment; care should be focused on keeping me comfortable and relieving symptoms, without the goal of extending my life. ("Keep me comfortable.")

Selective treatment: I would like to receive medical treatments **selectively**. Decisions should be based on my wishes and values, considering both the possibility of extending my life and the quality of my life. ("It depends.")

Maximum treatment: I am asking for all available treatment, with the goal of allowing me to live as long as possible. ("Do everything.")

Please review the following care situations and mark a point on the continuum (scale) that best describes the treatment approach that you would want if you were in that situation. *You do not need to answer every question and you may write in anything specific that you want your surrogate to know.*

A. Worsening of chronic physical illness

A **chronic illness** is one that lasts over a long period of time. A person may experience periods of improvement and periods of being sicker; the condition usually **cannot** be cured or reversed and may or may not be terminal.

A chronic illness may cause pain, trouble with breathing, or loss of mobility. Some examples of chronic illness include heart failure, severe arthritis, severe lung disease, paralysis due to a stroke, kidney failure and untreatable pain.

Sometimes chronic illness can become progressively worse and require multiple tests and frequent treatments.

If my chronic illness were to become progressively worse and threaten my life, I would want:

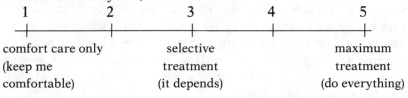

1	2	3	4	5

comfort care only   selective   maximum
(keep me   treatment   treatment
comfortable)   (it depends)   (do everything)

Comments:
_____
_____

B. Acute and chronic illness

A person with a chronic illness like the examples above may also develop an acute illness in addition to the chronic illness. An **acute illness** is one which is normally relatively short and has a good likelihood of being cured or reversed by appropriate medical care; it is not usually terminal. Examples of acute illness are pneumonia, urinary infection, or gastroenteritis (stomach distress). The evaluation and treatment of an acute illness may require blood tests or other tests, intravenous fluids, antibiotics and other treatments.

If my chronic illness were to become progressively worse and threaten my life, I would want:

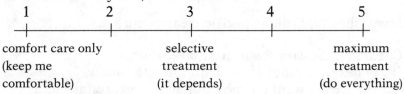

1	2	3	4	5

comfort care only   selective   maximum
(keep me   treatment   treatment
comfortable)   (it depends)   (do everything)

Comments:
_____
_____

C. Cognitive impairment

Cognition refers to the ability to think clearly; thinking or mental abilities include skills such as remembering, being aware of one's surroundings, exercising judgment and behaving appropriately. Cognitive impairment may result from many sources; two of the most common are Alzheimer's Disease and stroke.

If I become **cognitively impaired**, and develop medical problems, I would want:

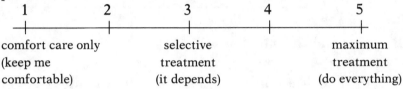

1	2	3	4	5
comfort care only (keep me comfortable)		selective treatment (it depends)		maximum treatment (do everything)

Comments:

_____

_____

D. Specific treatments

Some people have definite feelings regarding specific medical treatments. The following section allows you to let your surrogate know any wishes you might have as to whether you would definitely want, or definitely *not* want a particular treatment, or if you would want it only in specific circumstances.

My wishes regarding **specific treatments** are:

Cardio-pulmonary Resuscitation (CPR)*
If my heart or lungs should stop functioning:
_____ I would want cardio-pulmonary resuscitation.
_____ I would not want cardio-pulmonary resuscitation.
_____ I'm not sure.

Comments: _____

*It is very important that you discuss this with your physician.

Respirator (breathing by machine, through a tube in the throat) If I am unable to breathe independently:
_____ I **would** want to be placed on a respirator.
_____ I would **not** want to be placed on a respirator.
_____ I would want to be placed on a respirator, but would want this treatment discontinued if my physician judges that it is not meeting the treatment goals for which it was intended.
_____ I'm not sure.

Comments:_____

Artificial Nutrition and Hydration (feeding tube)
If I am unable to take food and/or fluids by mouth:
_____ I would want artificial nutrition and/or hydration (feeding tube).
_____ I would not want artificial nutrition and/or hydration (feeding tube).
_____ I would want this treatment tried, but discontinued if my physician judges that it is not meeting the treatment goals for which it was intended.
_____ I'm not sure.

Comments:_____

Surgery
If I develop a condition for which my physician presents surgery as an option:
_____ I **would** want surgery.
_____ I would **not** want surgery.
_____ I would want surgery only if the goal of surgery were to provide comfort or alleviate pain.
_____ I'm not sure.

Comments (please mention any preferences you have about specific surgical procedures): _____

_____

_____

Diagnostic Procedures
If my physician suggests invasive diagnostic procedures or
    tests (beyond routine blood tests and x-rays):
_____ I **would** want such tests.
_____ I would **not** want such tests.
_____ I would want such tests if my physician felt that the
    results would provide information which would be
    helpful in providing comfort or alleviating pain.
_____ I'm not sure.

Comments: _____

Hospitalization
If my physician judges that I have a condition for which s/
    he would recommend transfer to a hospital:
_____ I **would** want to be hospitalized.
_____ I would **not** want to be hospitalized.
_____ I would want to be hospitalized only if it were neces-
    sary in order to provide comfort or alleviate pain.
_____ I'm not sure.

Comments: _____

Dialysis (cleaning the blood by machine several times a
    week) If my kidneys cease to function and my physi-
    cian recommends dialysis:
_____ I **would** want dialysis.
_____ I would **not** want dialysis.
_____ I'm not sure.

Comments: _____

Other
(please specify other treatments about which you would
like to give instructions):

_____

_____

_____

Recording of this Document
Although this document is between you and your surro-
gate, and is not binding upon your physician, the informa-
tion within it could help your doctor to give guidance to
your surrogate should you become unable to make your
own decisions. Also, placing it in your medical record will
ensure that your surrogate always has access to this infor-
mation. However, this is your choice, so please indicate
your preference here:

_____ I would like this document included in my medical
       record.
_____ I would not like this document included in my medi-
       cal record.

**_

To my surrogate:
I am grateful for your willingness to help ensure that decisions regarding my care will reflect my values and goals. I
know that I cannot possibly anticipate every situation
which might occur, and I trust that you will do your best to
make decisions based on what you know of my values and
goals; this is all I ask of you.

_____   _____

Signature of resident/patient   Date

I have read and understand the above:

_____   _____

Signature of Surrogate   Date

Appendix V

Suggested Readings

NOTE: The following list of suggested additional readings is highly selective. It is restricted to books, reports, manuals, and articles that either (a) are seminal or foundational substantive or informational contributions to the modern literature regarding medical decisionmaking for the seriously ill or (b) provide particular insights into the ethical and legal issues connected to medical decisionmaking, advance medical directives, and operationalization of the Patient Self-Determination Act as those issues arise in the institutional or community-based long-term care context.

Books, Reports, and Manuals

Agich, G. J. (1993). *Autonomy in Long Term Care.* New York: Oxford University Press.

Cantor, N. L. (1993). *Advance Directives and the Pursuit of Death with Dignity.* Bloomington, IN: Indiana University Press.

Choice in Dying, Inc. (1991). *Advance Directive Protocols and the Patient Self-Determination Act.* New York: Author.

Choice in Dying, Inc. (1992, March). *Advance Directives and Community Education: A Manual for Institutional Caregivers.* New York: Author.

Glick, H. R. (1992). The Right to Die: Policy Innovation and Its Consequences. New York: Columbia University Press.

Hastings Center. (1987). Guidelines on the Termination of Life-Sustaining Treatment and the Care of the Dying. Briarcliff Manor, NY: Hastings Center.

Hill, T. P., & Shirley, D. (1992). A Good Death: Taking More Control at the End of Your Life. Reading, MA: Addison-Wesley Publishing Company, Inc.

Hofland, B. F. (Ed.) (1988, June). Autonomy and Long Term Care [Special Supplement]. Gerontologist, 28.

Hofland, B. F. (Ed.) (1990). Autonomy and Long-Term-Care Practice [Special Supplement]. Generations, 14.

Kapp, M. B. (1992). Geriatrics and the Law: Patient Rights and Professional Responsibilities (2d ed.) New York: Springer Publishing Company.

Kilner, J. F. (1992). Life on the Line: Ethics, Aging, Ending Patients' Lives, and Allocating Vital Resources. Grand Rapids, MI: William B. Eerdmans Publishing Company.

Logue, B. J. (1993). Last Rights: Death Control and the Elderly in America. New York: Lexington Books.

Miles, S. M., & Gomez, C. F. (1989). Protocols for Elective Use of Life-sustaining Treatments. New York: Springer Publishing Company.

Monagle, J. F., & Thomasma, D. C. (1993). Medical Ethics: Policies, Protocols, Guidelines, and Programs. Frederick, MD: Aspen Publishers, Inc.

Moody, H. R. (1992). Ethics in an Aging Society. Baltimore: Johns Hopkins University Press.

National Health Lawyers Association. (1991). The Patient Self-Determination Directory & Resource Guide. Washington, DC: Author.

Office of Technology Assessment (1987, July). Life-Sustaining Technologies and the Elderly (OTA–BA–306). Washington, DC: U.S. Government Printing Office.

President's Commission for the Study of Ethical Problems in Biomedical and Behavioral Research. Deciding to Forego Life-Sustaining Treatment: Ethical, Medical and Legal Issues in Treatment Decisions. Washington, DC: U.S. Government Printing Office.

Quill, T. E. (1993). Death and Dignity: Making Choices and Taking Charge. New York: W. W. Norton & Company.

Ross, J. R., Glaser, J. W., Rasinski-Gregory, D., Gibson, J. M., & Bayley, C. (1993). *Health Care Ethics Committees: The Next Generation*. Chicago: American Hospital Publishing.
Urofsky, M.I. (1993). *Letting Go: Death, Dying & The Law*. New York: Charles Scribner's Sons.

Articles

American Medical Association Council on Scientific Affairs and Council on Ethical and Judicial Affairs (1990). Persistent vegetative state and the decision to withdraw or withhold life support. *Journal of the American Medical Association, 263*, 426–430.
American Medical Association Council on Ethical and Judicial Affairs (1992). Decisions near the end of life. *Journal of the American Medical Association, 267*, 2229–2233.
Besdine, R. W. (1983, October). Decisions to withhold treatment from nursing home residents. *Journal of the American Geriatrics Society, 31*, 602–606.
Cogen, R., Patterson, B., Clavin, S., Cogen, J., Landsberg, L., & Posner, J. (1992, September). Surrogate decision-maker preferences for medical care of severely demented nursing home patients. *Archives of Internal Medicine, 152*, 1885–1888.
Cohen, C. B. (1992, Winter). Avoiding cloudcuckooland in ethics committee case review: Matching models to issues and concerns. *Law, Medicine & Health Care, 20*, 294–299.
Cohen-Mansfield, J., Rabinovich, B. A., Lipson, S., Fein, A., Gerber, B., Weisman, S., & Pawlson, L. G. (1991, February). The decision to execute a durable power of attorney for health care and preferences regarding the utilization of life-sustaining treatments in nursing home residents. *Archives of Internal Medicine, 151*, 289–294.
Collopy, B., Dubler, N., & Zuckerman, C. (1990, March-April). The ethics of home care: Autonomy and accommodation. *Hastings Center Report, 20*, No. 2: Supp. 1–16.
Collopy, B., Boyle, P., & Jennings, B. (1991, March-April). New directions in nursing home ethics. *Hastings Center Report, 21*, No. 21 Supp. 1–16.
Connaway, N. I. (1985). Relying on the living will in home health care. *Home Healthcare Nurse, 3*, 42–45.
Diamond, E. L., Jernigan, J. A., Moseley, R. A., Messina, V., &

McKeown, R. A. (1989, October). Decision-making ability and advance directive preferences in nursing home patients and proxies. *Gerontologist, 29*, 622–626.

Dubler, N. N. (1990, Fall). Refusals of medical care in the home setting. *Law, Medicine & Health Care, 18*, 227–233.

Emanuel, L. (1991, December). The health care directive: Learning how to draft advance care documents. *Journal of the American Geriatrics Society, 39*, 1221–1228.

Henderson, M. (1990, August). Beyond the living will. *Gerontologist, 30*, 480–485.

Johnson, S. (1991, September-October). PSDA in the nursing home. *Hastings Center Report, 21*, S3–4.

Kayser-Jones, J. (1990, August). The use of nasogastric feeding tubes in nursing homes: Patient, family and health care provider perspectives. *Gerontologist, 30*, 469–479.

Lurie, N., Pheley, A. M., Miles, S. H., & Bannick-Mohrland, S. (1992, December). Attitudes toward discussing life-sustaining treatments in extended care facility patients. *Journal of the American Geriatrics Society, 40*, 1205–1208.

Madson, S. K. (1993, February). Patient Self-Determination Act: Implications for long term care. *Journal of Gerontological Nursing, 19*, 15–18.

McIntyre, K. M. (1992, February). Shepherding the patient's right to self-determination: The physician's dawning role. *Archives of Internal Medicine, 152*, 259–261.

Meisel, A. (1992, December). The legal consensus about foregoing life-sustaining treatment: Its status and its prospects. *Kennedy Institute of Ethics Journal, 2*, 309–345.

Meisel, A. *The Right to Die* (1989, supplemented annually). New York: John Wiley and Sons.

Michelson, C., Mulvihill, M., Hsu, M. A., & Olson, E. (1991, June). Eliciting medical care preferences from nursing home residents. *Gerontologist, 31*, 358–363.

Miles, S. H., Bannick-Mohrland, S., & Lurie, N. (1990, Summer). Advance-treatment planning discussions with nursing home residents: Pilot experience with simulated interviews. *Journal of Clinical Ethics, 1*, 108–112.

Miller, T., & Cugliari, A. M. (1990, August). Withdrawing and withholding treatment: Policies in long-term care facilities. *Gerontologist, 30*, 462–468.

Olson, E., Chichin, E. R., Libon, L. S., Martico-Greenfield, T.,

Neufeld, R., & Mulvihill, M. (1993, April). A center on ethics in long-term care. *Gerontologist, 33,* 269–274.

Rango, N. (1985, June). The nursing home resident with dementia: Clinical care, ethics, and policy implications. *Annals of Internal Medicine, 102,* 835–841.

Refolo, M. A. (1992). The Patient Self-Determination Act of 1990: Health care's own *Miranda. Journal of Contemporary Health Law and Policy, 8,* 455–471.

Rouse, F. (1988, Summer). Living wills in the long-term care facility. *Journal of Long-Term Care Administration, 16,* 14–19.

Uhlmann, R. F., Clark, H., Pearlman, R. A., Downs, J. C., Addison, J. H., & Haining, R. G. (1987, June). Medical management decisions in nursing home patients. *Annals of Internal Medicine, 106,* 879–885.

Von Preyss-Friedman, S. M., Uhlmann, R. F., & Cain, K. C. (1992, January-February). Physicians' attitudes toward tube feeding chronically ill nursing home patients. *Journal of General Internal Medicine, 7,* 46–51.

Wolf, S. M. (1991). Ethics committees and due process: Nesting rights in a community of caring. *Maryland Law Review, 50,* 798–858.

Wood, J. S. (1986, August). Nursing home care. *Clinics in Geriatric Medicine, 2,* 601–615.

Index

213

Springer Publishing Company

LONG-TERM CARE CASE MANAGEMENT
Design and Evaluation

Robert A. Applebaum, PhD and **Carol D. Austin**, PhD

Distills essential features and basic concepts, spotlighting the main components of a case management program and presenting a logically organized description of how such programs may differ given a set number of variables. Highlights pros and cons of numerous design features.

Contents:

I: Designing Case Management: Basic Concepts • Components of Case Management • How Program Variables Affect Case Management Service Delivery • Case Mangement Design Options

II: Evaluating and Assuring the Quality of Case Managed Care: Evaluation and Quality Assurance of Case Management: An Overview • Assessing the Outcomes of Case Management Practice

III: Past Experiences and Future Challenges: The Evolution of Case Management Service Delivery • Issues in Planning a Case Management Program

1990   192pp   0-8261-6430-7   hardcover

AN ORIENTATION MANUAL FOR LONG-TERM CARE FACILITIES
A Program for Developing and Retaining
Vital Employees, Second Edition

Joan M. Iannone, MSN, RN, C, and **Margaret Gorely Bye**, RN, EdD

This is a complete "how-to" manual that meets all federal requirements for orientation to long-term care facilities.

Partial Contents:

I: Theory and Practice for the Staff. • Development Coordinator • Adult Education Principles and Practice • Teaching the Learner with Low-Literacy Skills

II: An Orientation Program for Long-Term Care. • Organizational Structure and Philosphy • Personnel • Facility Tour • Concepts of Aging • Body Mechanics • Resident Rights • Communication Skills • Fire Safety

III: What Next? Articulation from a General Orientation to a Departmental Orientation or a Nurse Aide Training Program

1993   216pp   0-8261-8280-1   hardcover

536 Broadway, New York, NY 10012-3955 • (212) 431-4370 • Fax (212) 941-7842

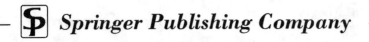
Springer Publishing Company

JOURNAL OF LONG TERM HOME HEALTH CARE

The PRIDE Institute Journal

Editor: **Philip W. Brickner**, M.D.

Editorial Board: **James Paul Firman**, EdD.,
Mathy D. Mezey, Ed.D., R.N., F.A.A.N.,
Bart Price, C.P.A., **Linda Keen Scharer**, M.U.P.,
Rolando A. Thorne, M.P.H.

Beginning in 1994, Springer Publishing Company proudly added the former PRIDE Institute Journal to its Library of Long-Term Care. This essential quarterly provides articles that present research, analyze current issues, and report on programs in the long term home health care field.

Each issue features papers that offer detailed analysis of topics in the diverse arenas of long term home health care, forecast developments, and provide readers with an enhanced perspective. Each issue includes an editorial, book reviews, and a list of books recieved. The Editorial and Consulting Boards, consisting of distinguished specialists in the field, have provided special issues such as "Ethical Issues in Long Term Care","Homeless Elders: Prevention and Intervention", "Alcohol Use and Abuse in the Aged","Cultural Competence in the Care Of Elderly Chinese Persons", and "Caring for the Difficult Patient at Home".

Sample Contents:

Mechanisms of Falls in Community Residing Older Persons, R. Tideiksaar • Recognizing and Responding to Elder Maltreatment, H. Ramsey-Klawsnik • Youth Exchanging With Seniors: A Rural Texas Program, S. H. Boyd, B. L. Stout & K. Volanty • Financial Self-Sufficiency Through Operating Revenue at Two Adult Day Centers, B. V. Reifler, et al. • Assessing the Needs of Persons of Advanced Age: The Weston, Massachusettes Council on Aging "Over 80" Outreach Survey, S. S. Earle • Commentary:Continuing Care Retirement Communities, D. Schwartz

ISSN 1072-4281 • *4 issues annually*

536 Broadway, New York, NY 10012-3955 • (212) 431-4370 • Fax (212) 941-7842

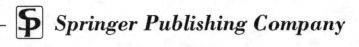
PROBLEM BEHAVIORS IN LONG-TERM CARE:
Recognition, Diagnosis, and Treatment

Peggy A. Szwabo, RN, ACSW, C-CS, and
George T. Grossberg, MD, Editors

Foreword: Rosalie A. Kane, DSW

A practical guide to common problems facing geriatric nurses, social workers, and physicians in their contact with the elderly.

Partial Contents:

Special Populations in Extended Care Facilities, *M.S. Harper* • Problem Behaviors Among Younger Adult Nursing Home Residents, *J.C. Romeis* • Recognition and Treatment of Depression in the Nursing Home, *J. Manepalli and G.T. Grossberg* • Eating and Nutritional Disorders, *A.J. Silver* • Management of Pain in the Elderly, *R.C. Tait* • Wandering: Assessment and Intervention, *D.L. Algase* • Use of Physical Restraints and Options, *H.W. Lach* • Special Care Units, *S. Bass, et al.*

Nurse's Book Society Selection
1992   320pp   0-8261-7820-0   hardcover

ETHNIC ELDERLY AND LONG-TERM CARE

Charles M. Barresi, PhD, and
Donald E. Stull, PhD, Editors

This multidisciplinary volume spans family caregiving at home to institutional care and examines various model programs designed especially for the ethnic elderly.

Partial Contents:

Ethnicity and Long-Term Care: An Overview, *C.M. Barresi & D.E. Stull* • Ethnic Variations in Measurement of Physical Health Status, *E. Bastida & G. Gonzalez* • Ethnicity and Minority Issues in Family Caregiving to Rural Black Elders, *J.B. Wood & T.T.H. Wan* • Self-Care Practices of Black Elders, *L.H. Davis & B.F. McGadney* • Functional Abilities of Chinese and Korean Elders in Congregate Housing, *E.S.H. Yu, et al.* •Long-Term Care of Older American Indians, *S.M. Manson* • Adaptation to Institutional Life Among Polish, Jewish, and Western European Elderly, *E. Kahana, et al.* •   On Lok's Model: Managed Long-Term Care, *C. Van Steenberg, et al.* • Hispanic Elderly: Policy Issues in Long-Term Care, *C.G. Lacayo* • Ethnic Seniors' Preferences for Long-Term Care Services and Financing, *D.E. Stull*

1992 312pp 0-8261-7370-5 hardcover

536 Broadway, New York, NY 10012-3955 • (212) 431-4370 • Fax (212) 941-7842